Study Guide to Accompany

Maternal & Child Health Nursing

CARE OF THE CHILDBEARING & CHILDREARING FAMILY

REVISED REPRINT, FIFTH EDITION

Study Guide to Accompany

Maternal & Child Health Nursing

CARE OF THE CHILDBEARING & CHILDREARING FAMILY

REVISED REPRINT, FIFTH EDITION

Prepared by

Joyce Young Johnson, Ph.D., R.N.

Resource Nurse/Nursing Service
Crawford Long Hospital of Emory University
Adjunct Faculty
School of Nursing
Georgia State University
Atlanta, Georgia

Edna Boyd-Davis, R.N., B.S.N., M.N.

Assistant Professor
School of Nursing and Allied Health
Atlanta, Georgia Unit
Tuskegee University
Atlanta, Georgia
Clinical Nurse Specialist
Hughes Spalding Children's Hospital
Atlanta, Georgia
Lieutenant Colonel
Army Nurse Corps
United States Army
Fort Gordon, Georgia

Visit the Lippincott's NursingCenter Website
http://www.nursingcenter.com

Visit the Lippincott Williams & Wilkins Website
http://www.lww.com

Wolters Kluwer Health | Lippincott Williams & Wilkins

Philadelphia • Baltimore • New York • London
Buenos Aires • Hong Kong • Sydney • Tokyo

Ancillary Editor: Audrey Lickwar
Compositor: Spearhead
Printer/Binder: Port City Press

ISBN 13: 978-0-7817-8708-6
ISBN 10: 0-7817-8708-4
7 6 5 4 3 2

To my husband Larry, my daughter Virginia, and my son Larry Jr. who make life worth living; in memory of my father, Riley H. Young Sr, and to my Mother, Dorothy Young, my sisters, brother, and best friends who have always supported and nurtured me and whose faith in me continues to motivate me.

Joyce Young Johnson

To my son Jakara Boyd Davis of whom I am so very proud.
To my father who always encouraged me to excel and to the memory of my mother and brother who taught me never to give up!
To my brother, Roy I. Mitchell, who teaches me the value of patience and to my friend, Gail Witsell Morrell, who is always there for me!

Edna Boyd-Davis

To our students, who are the reasons we do what we do.

Contributors to the Second Edition

Christine Hatch, R.N.
Stone Mountain, Georgia
Chapter 23: Nursing Care of the Newborn and Family
Chapter 30: The Family With a Toddler

Phyllis Prather Hicks, R.N., B.S.N.
Harrisburg Area Community College
Harrisburg, Pennsylvania
Chapter 35: The Effects of Hospitalization on Children and Their Families
Chapter 36: Health Teaching With Children
Chapter 37: Nursing Care of the Hospitalized Child and Family: Diagnostic and Therapeutic Techniques

Anita Price, R.N.
Buford, Georgia
Chapter 21: The Woman Who Develops a Complication During Labor and Birth

Anthelyn Jean Smith Temple, M.S.N., R.N.
University of South Alabama
Mobile, Alabama
Chapter 55: Nursing Care of the Family in Crisis: Child and Domestic Abuse
Chapter 56: The Family Coping with Long-Term or Fatal Illness

Contributors to the First Edition

Geraldine C. Fells, R.N., M.A., M.S.
Clayton State College
Morrow, Georgia

Phyllis Prather Hicks, R.N., B.S.N.
Harrisburg Area Community College
Harrisburg, Pennsylvania

Brenda Raper, R.N., C.N.P.
Fulton County Health Department
Atlanta, Georgia

Elaine Embrack Ridgeway, R.N., M.S.N., C.I.C.
Rockdale Hospital
Conyers, Georgia

Gayle Russo, R.N., M.N., C.D.E., A.N.P.
Emory University
Atlanta, Georgia

Preface

This student workbook is designed to accompany the fifth edition of *Maternal and child Health Nursing: Care of the Childbearing and Childrearing Family* by Adele Pillitteri. The workbook material directly addresses the units in the textbook and provides exercises to assist the student in learning important terms and concepts. Some anatomy, physiology, and pathophysiology concepts are addressed; however, a major focus is the role nurses play in helping the nation meet health goals by providing quality maternal-newborn and child health nursing care. The use of the nursing process to address the physiologic and psychosocial needs of the client and family in a holistic and culturally appropriate manner is addressed by the questions in this workbook.

The workbook is divided into chapters that correlate with those in the text. Generally, each chapter in the study guide contains the following elements:

Chapter Overview: A summary of the content in the textbook chapter.
Learning Objectives: A list of learning goals that you will be able to meet after you read the textbook and work through the exercises in this study guide.
Key terms: Identify the major terms the students should be familiar with after completing the chapter.
Section one: Identification of key terms and concepts, which includes exercises to assist you in mastering content. These exercises may vary but will include such items as matching, true or false, and completion and short answer. A brief description of these item types follows:
Matching: Questions that most often address the definitions of key terms or the meaning of key concepts
True or False: Questions that are answered by knowing whether the statement is true or false. In the answer key, the false statements are corrected so you will know what part of the statement was in error and what information is accurate.
Completion: Questions that require you to supply the missing information. The answers may be as short as one or a few words or as long as a short paragraph. Where a more lengthy answer is required, several lines are provided. Where answers of one or a few words are required, a single line is provided.
A new feature in the study guide is the inclusion of the following sections:
NCLEX Preparation: Various multiple-choice questions that focus on nursing care or other clinical information.
NCLEX Preparation for alternative items: Include completion, multiple correct answer items in which you must select all that apply, and items in which you must rank order information, prioritize data, or identify a structure.
Inquiry and Exploration: Includes a case study and exercises to help you apply the information learned through critical inquiry and critical exploration while answering questions designed specifically to allow you to analyze client situations while applying essential concepts. These learning exercises provide individual and clinical activities that will broaden your knowledge and understanding of the content covered in the chapter.

The instructor may assign an entire workbook chapter or parts of the chapter, as needed. We hope that both the text and workbook provide the student with an opportunity to fully explore and learn about the important concepts of maternal-newborn and child health nursing.

Joyce Young Johnson, Ph.D., R.N.
Edna Boyd-Davis, R.N., B.S.N., M.N.

Acknowledgments

We would like to thank everyone at Lippincott Williams & Wilkins who helped throughout the production of this edition of the study guide. We would above all like to thank Doris Wray for her support and assistance and Elizabeth Nieginski and Claudia Vaughn for their guidance during the production of this manuscript. We would also like to thank Gail Witsell Morrell, LaGretta Walton, and Troycia Webb for their valuable service in the preparation of this manuscript.

Contents

UNIT I

Maternal and Child Health Nursing Practice

CHAPTER 1

A Framework for Maternal and Child Health Nursing

CHAPTER OVERVIEW

Chapter 1 presents an overview of maternal and child health nursing. The use of nursing process, nursing research, and nursing theory in the provision of quality care is discussed. The standards of nursing practice and the varied roles assumed by nurses in maternal and child health nursing are also explored.

LEARNING OBJECTIVES

After mastering the content in this chapter, you should be able to do the following:

1. Identify the goals and philosophy of maternal and child health nursing.
2. Describe the evolution, scope, and professional roles for nurses in maternal and child health nursing.
3. Define common statistical terms used in the field, such as infant and maternal mortality.
4. Discuss the implications of the common standards of maternal and child health nursing and the health goals for the nation for maternal and child health nursing practice.
5. Discuss the interplay of nursing process, evidence-based practice, and nursing theory as they relate to the future of maternal and child health nursing practice.
6. Use critical thinking to identify areas of care that could benefit from additional nursing research, or application of evidence-based practice.
7. Apply concepts of family-centered care to maternal-child nursing
8. Integrate knowledge of trends in maternal and child health care with the nursing process to achieve an understanding of quality maternal and child health nursing care.

KEY TERMS

clinical nurse specialist
evidence-based practice
family nurse practitioner
fertility rate
maternal and child health nursing
maternal-newborn nursing
mortality rate
neonatal nurse practitioner
neonate
nurse-midwife
nursing research
pediatric nurse practitioner
puerperium
scope of practice
women's health practitioner

■ Mastering the Information

MATCHING

Match the terms in Column I with a definition, example, or related statement from Column II. Place the letter corresponding to the answer in the space provided.

COLUMN I

1. _____ Guidelines developed by the American Nurses Association and Association of Women's Health, Obstetric, and Neonatal Nurses
2. _____ Prompt diagnosis and treatment of illness using interventions that will return the client to wellness most rapidly
3. _____ Controlled investigation of problems with implications for nursing practice
4. _____ Care of a woman before conception and through pregnancy, and care of the child prenatally, from birth and the neonatal period, and from infancy through adolescence
5. _____ The 6-week period following childbirth; the "fourth trimester"

6. _____ Use of research as a foundation of action
7. _____ Education of clients to be aware of good health through teaching and role modeling
8. _____ The promotion and maintenance of optimal family health to ensure cycles of optimal childbearing and childrearing

COLUMN II

a. Maternal and child nursing
b. Health promotion
c. Nursing research
d. Primary goal of maternal and child health nursing
e. Health restoration
f. Standards of maternal and child health nursing practice
g. Puerperium
h. Evidence-based practice

SHORT ANSWER

Supply the missing term or the information requested.

1. Discuss two of six trends in maternal and child health nursing care and the associated implications for nurses.
2. Explain the effect that shorter hospital stays will have on client care planning for a child during the postoperative period, particularly on client and family teaching.
3. Discuss methods of promoting empowerment of parents and children in the health care setting.

■ Applying Your Knowledge

CASE STUDY

Chin Won, age 26, presents at the community health center in her last trimester of pregnancy for her initial prenatal care visit. She is found to have an elevated blood pressure and excessive swelling in her legs and feet. The fetus appears small on the sonogram.

1. What are some reasons that early prenatal care might have helped to decrease Chin Won's risk for maternal mortality and perinatal mortality?
2. What measures might the nurse take to ensure that Chin Won's care is family-centered?
3. How might cultural assessment be beneficial when planning with Chin Won for health restoration and maintenance throughout the pregnancy and puerperium?
4. How would the plan of care look if Chin Won were a single woman, a working mother, or a teen?

CRITICAL INQUIRY EXERCISE

1. Write a brief statement on your opinion regarding termination of pregnancy when the woman is at risk from the pregnancy and the fetus is healthy.
2. Prepare a plan for establishing an environment in which a hospitalized child can maintain a sense of parenting and family security. Include discussions of room appearance, visiting arrangements, care schedule, and input into care activities.

CRITICAL EXPLORATION

Examine the policy at a local maternal-child care facility regarding the procedure a nurse must follow if she suspects that a woman and her children are victims of an abusive male family member.

■ Practicing for NCLEX

MULTIPLE-CHOICE QUESTIONS

Circle the letter that corresponds to the best answer for each question.

1. Maternal mortality is defined as the number of:
   A. fetal deaths occurring as a result of maternal negligence during pregnancy.
   B. maternal deaths per 100,000 live births occurring as a direct result of the reproductive process.
   C. pregnancies per 1,000 women that result in maternal death.
   D. fetal deaths (fetus weight over 500 g) per 1,000 live births resulting in maternal death.

2. A newly admitted client expresses a wish to continue taking the herbal medicine she brought from home to help relieve her abdominal pain. Which of the following would be an appropriate reply?
   A. "You shouldn't believe in alternative therapies; they don't work as well as modern medications."
   B. "The doctor won't like it if you take any medication other than that prescribed."
   C. "You can take the herbal medication, but only after you've taken the prescribed medications I give you."
   D. "We have to check the herbal treatment to be sure it doesn't interfere with prescribed medications."

3. Which of the following represents an important implication for nursing related to the regionalization of pediatric care?
   A. Being away from home represents a fun adventure to children, so the nurse must ensure that the child takes health care seriously.
   B. Having the family members in a different city will allow for better bonding between the child and the hospital staff.
   C. Regionalization allows the nurse to isolate the child from parental overprotectiveness, which might slow development.
   D. The nurse has the responsibility to see that children and parents feel as welcome in the regional center as they would in a small hospital.

4. Since health care consumers are increasingly discriminating in their demands, which of the following would be most effective in facilitating consumer empowerment by the maternal-child health nurse?
   A. Allow minimal input from the client and family members into the planning of care to prevent excessive interference.
   B. Keep family members informed and help them make decisions about their child's care.
   C. Limit family visitation to prevent collaboration with the client and discovery of minor errors in care.
   D. Remind the client and family members that in the hospital setting, the nurse is in charge.

5. Which statement is an accurate description of an expanded role for nurses in maternal-child health?
   A. Clinical nurse specialists are prepared at the baccalaureate degree level and are capable of independent care of children.
   B. If a pediatric nurse practitioner (PNP) determines that a child has a major illness, the PNP can independently prescribe appropriate medication.
   C. Nurse-midwives can assume full responsibility for the care and management of women with uncomplicated pregnancies.
   D. Pediatric nurse practitioners are registered nurses who are usually prepared at the associate degree level.

ALTERNATE FORMAT QUESTIONS

Fill in the Blank

Supply the missing term or the information requested.

1. The ______ ______ ______ is skilled in the care of the newborn, both ill and well.
2. The nurse must understand the ______________ of practice, which is the range of services and care that may be provided by the nurse based on state requirements.

Multiple-Answer Multiple Choice

Circle the letter(s) corresponding to the appropriate answer(s). Select all that apply.

1. The leading causes of neonatal infant mortality are:
   A. Prematurity
   B. Low birthweight
   C. Congenital anomalies
   D. Gestational diabetes
   E. Malnutrition

2. Which of the following are examples of the implications for nursing as related to the trends and concerns regarding health care costs?
   A. The average American cannot afford to hire a nurse practitioner instead of a physician to provide less expensive but more comprehensive family health care.
   B. Nurses must become more cost conscious about supplies and services and help reduce cost while maintaining quality care.
   C. Health care is less expensive today because most families have begun to participate in health promotion activities using primary care nurses.
   D. Lack of financial ability to pay is a major reason for women not seeking and obtaining prenatal care.
   E. Access to support from governmental programs has eliminated most of the problems associated with absence of prenatal care.

CHAPTER 2

The Childbearing and Childrearing Family and Community

CHAPTER OVERVIEW

Chapter 2 provides a description of the family and how nursing is involved in family-centered care. The types of families and family tasks are described according to Duvall and Miller (1990). The importance of providing nursing care that addresses families at their level of understanding, as indicated by their stage of development, is well demonstrated. This chapter challenges the student to use the community assessment tool to assist him or her in determining the relation of the family to the community. The student is instructed to use the outcome criteria to formulate a nursing plan of care. A case study is presented to provide the student with the principles of parenting as they relate to the adopted child.

LEARNING OBJECTIVES

After mastering the content in this chapter, you should be able to do the following:

1. Describe family structure, function, and family roles.
2. Assess a family for structure and healthy function.
3. Formulate nursing diagnoses related to family health.
4. Develop expected outcome criteria to help a family to achieve optimal health.
5. Plan health teaching strategies, such as helping a family modify its lifestyle to adjust to pregnancy or accommodate an ill child.
6. Implement nursing care, such as teaching a family more effective wellness behaviors.
7. Evaluate outcome criteria for achievement and effectiveness of nursing care to be certain that outcomes goals have been achieved.
8. Identify National Health Goals related to the family and specific ways that nurses can help the nation achieve these goals.
9. Identify areas of care related to family nursing that could benefit from additional nursing research or the application of evidence-based practice.
10. Use critical thinking to analyze additional ways that nursing care can be family-centered or that client maternal care can better include family members.
11. Integrate knowledge of family nursing with the nursing process to promote quality maternal and child health nursing care.

KEY TERMS

community
ecomap
family
family of orientation
family of procreation
family theory
nursing genogram

■ Mastering the Information

MATCHING

Match the terms in Column II with a definition, example, or related statement from Column I. Place the letter corresponding to the answer in the space provided.

COLUMN I

1. _____ An important nursing role is health education concerning well-child care. The nurse should also assess the parents' ability to care for an infant with health problems.
2. _____ Accidents involving children are a major health concern, and growth and development needs and safety considerations are increased.
3. _____ Older family members are more likely to suffer from chronic and disabling conditions than are younger members.

4. _____ Members of the family work to obtain a mutually satisfying relationship, relate well to their families, and plan for parenthood.

5. _____ Accidents, homicide, and suicide are the major causes of death. The nurse has an important role in facilitating communication between family members and spends time counseling them on safety, proper care of and respect for firearms, and drug abuse.

COLUMN II

a. Family with adolescent children
b. Early childbearing family
c. Family with preschool children
d. The family in retirement
e. Marriage and the family

SHORT ANSWER

Supply the missing term or the information requested.

1. Parents may receive remuneration for their care; children in these families may feel very insecure. This type of family is called a ________ family.
2. Members are related by social values, are free choice-oriented, and/or may follow a charismatic leader. This type of family is called a ________________________ family.

■ Applying Your Knowledge

CASE STUDY

The nurse is counseling a family who is anticipating the adoption of a 6-year-old boy. The family is currently in the marriage stage of growth and development.

1. What rationale should the nurse use to formulate an approach when advising this family to visit a health care facility soon after the adopted child has arrived in the home?
2. How does the nurse explain why a larger percentage of adopted children may be put into a "high-risk" category for neurologic development?
3. What are some common factors that exist with parents who adopt children that may cause the parents to be less resilient when adjusting their lives to the presence of a new baby?
4. Why is it important for the adoptive parents to tell the child of his adoption as early as possible?
5. The adoption has been final for 6 months, and the family visits the community health center for a well-child preschool check-up. The parents state that the child exhibited defiant and hostile behaviors after being told of his adoption. How would the nurse analyze this behavior and give an explanation to the parents?

CRITICAL INQUIRY EXERCISE

1. Identify a patient in your clinical setting and use the family assessment tool to identify the various systems in his or her community.
2. Use the results to create an ecomap (diagram depicting the relationship between the family and the community).

CRITICAL EXPLORATION

Select a patient you are caring for in the clinical setting and create a nursing care plan for him or her, including an assessment of the family and community. State the nursing diagnosis found in making your assessment, and provide the appropriate nursing orders.

■ Practicing for NCLEX

MULTIPLE-CHOICE QUESTIONS

Circle the letter that corresponds to the best answer for each question.

1. Which of the following would be representative of a goal related to achieving healthy family and community life?
   A. Maintain the baseline positive for blood lead levels.
   B. Work with families with financial management.
   C. Lower the amount of physical abuse directed toward women.
   D. Support gay rights activists.

2. Which of the following best describes family nursing?
   A. Concentrates on the family as the client
   B. Concentrates on the individual as the client
   C. Concentrates on the family point of view
   D. Concentrates on the individual's point of view

3. Which of the following is a characteristic of the single-parent family?
   A. Provides support to family members due to its small size
   B. Involves reconstitution support and increased security
   C. Represents 50% to 60% of families with school-age children
   D. Uses family resources to provide temporary psychosocial comfort

ALTERNATE FORMAT QUESTIONS

Fill in the Blank

Supply the missing term or the information requested.

1. How well a family works together and meets any crisis depends on its structure and __________.
2. Homosexual unions in which children may be added to the family by artificial insemination or adoption represent a __________________ family.
3. A family of orientation is the family one is born into, and a family of __________________ is one the person establishes.

Multiple-Answer Multiple Choice

Circle the letter(s) corresponding to the appropriate answer(s). Select all that apply.

1. List the tasks discussed in your text according to Duvall and Miller (1990). Circle all that apply.
   A. Physical maintenance
   B. Socialization of family members
   C. Directions and marriage counseling recommendations
   D. Support as counsel during divorce
   E. Division of labor

2. Which of the following correctly describes a dyad family unit?
   A. Husband
   B. Wife
   C. Male child
   D. Woman
   E. Man

CHAPTER 3

Sociocultural Aspects of Maternal and Child Health Nursing

CHAPTER OVERVIEW

Chapter 3 provides the student with a fundamental understanding of cultural differences and exercises to assist the student in identifying behaviors that are culture-specific while respecting the individuality of all persons. A case study is presented to assist the student in planning for nutritional support as it relates to culture. The critical thinking exercises include the formulation of a nursing care plan.

LEARNING OBJECTIVES

After mastering the content in this chapter, you should be able to do the following:

1. Describe ways that sociocultural influences affect maternal and child health nursing care.
2. Assess a family for sociocultural influences that might influence the way it responds to childbearing and childrearing.
3. Formulate nursing diagnoses related to culturally appropriate aspects of nursing care.
4. Develop outcomes to assist families who have specific cultural needs to thrive in their community.
5. Plan and implement nursing care that respects the sociocultural needs and wishes of families.
6. Evaluate outcomes for achievement of care.
7. Identify National Health Goals related to sociocultural considerations that nurses can help the nation achieve.
8. Identify areas of care related to sociocultural considerations that could benefit from additional nursing research or application of evidence-based practice.
9. Use critical thinking to analyze how the sociocultural aspects of care affect family functioning and develop ways to make nursing care more family-centered.
10. Integrate sociocultural aspects of care with the nursing process to achieve quality maternal and child health nursing care.

KEY TERMS

acculturation	norms
assimilation	pain threshold
cultural values	pain tolerance
culture	stereotyping
ethnicity	taboos
ethnocentrism	threshold sensation
mores	transcultural nursing

■ Mastering the Information

MATCHING

Match the terms in Column II with a definition, example, or related statement from Column I. Place the letter corresponding to the answer in the space provided.

COLUMN I

1. ______ Individual perception that one's own culture is superior to all others
2. ______ A view of the world and a set of traditions that a specific social group uses and transmits to the next generation
3. ______ A cultural group into which one was born
4. ______ Expectation of a set of behavioral characteristics from a group without regard to their individual characteristics
5. ______ The care of patients with cultural aspects as a guide to care
6. ______ Integration of cultural elements to enhance communication

COLUMN II

a. Culture
b. Transcultural nursing
c. Cultural competence
d. Stereotyping
e. Ethnocentrism
f. Ethnicity

TRUE OR FALSE

Indicate if the following statements are true or false by placing a "T" or "F" in the space provided.

_____ 1. The predominant culture in the United States stresses that everyone should be employed productively (the Protestant work ethic).

_____ 2. Some families may use trusted family members as a reference for health care rather than a physician.

■ Applying Your Knowledge

CASE STUDY

Tatiana Ochoa is a 30-year-old Mexican-American woman in her second trimester of pregnancy. She is visiting the clinic for a prenatal examination. The nurse finds that Mrs. Ochoa is anemic.

1. What approach will the nurse use to assess the source of Mrs. Ochoa's anemia?

2. What cultural practice related to nutrition may be responsible for the anemia?

3. What suggestions might the nurse offer to facilitate adequate nutritional intake to correct the anemia yet allow Mrs. Ochoa to assume the diet she prefers?

CRITICAL INQUIRY EXERCISE

1. Some hospitals have taken an active role to include cultural sensitivity in the care of patients and their families. Research the hospitals in your area to identify those who have telephone service agreements to assist families with language interpretation.

2. Collaborate with your classmates to create a mock nursing care plan for patients of an ethnic orientation who may be experiencing problems attending appointments or making the appointments on time.

CRITICAL EXPLORATION

Select a patient you are caring for in the clinical setting and create a nursing care plan for him or her, including an assessment of the family and community. State the nursing diagnosis found in making your assessment, and provide the appropriate nursing orders.

■ Practicing for NCLEX

MULTIPLE-CHOICE QUESTIONS

Circle the letter that corresponds to the best answer for each question.

1. Which of the following phrases best describes assimilation as related to sociocultural differences?
   A. An adoption of the most dominant culture's values and influences
   B. A loss of cultural expression as the customs of a dominant culture are taken on
   C. A family tradition practiced in future generations
   D. Placement of "labels" on groups of people according to their ethnic backgrounds

2. Select the statement that best describes the nuclear family.
   A. A family consisting of the mother, father, and children
   B. A family consisting of the mother, father, children, and grandparents
   C. A family consisting of the mother, father, children, aunts, uncles, and cousins
   D. A family consisting of the mother or father and children

3. In the 1800s large numbers of immigrants came to the United States from many different countries and gave up their native country's traditions and values. Which of the following is the common explanation for the actions of these immigrants?
   A. Each culture found the American culture and beliefs to be equal or superior to their own.
   B. The immigrants feared the Americans and participated in the American culture to avoid cruelty and punishment.
   C. The immigrants joined the American "melting pot."
   D. Immigrants who did not take on the American culture were placed in lower socioeconomic groups.

ALTERNATE FORMAT QUESTIONS

Fill in the Blank

Supply the missing term or the information requested.

1. The term ——— commonly refers to people who speak Spanish as their primary language.
2. ————— avoid making direct eye contact with another individual during a conversation as a form of respect.

Multiple-Answer Multiple Choice

Circle the letter(s) corresponding to the appropriate answer(s). Select all that apply.

1. Which of the following strategies would be helpful in recognizing cultural influences on pain management?
   A. Using an assessment tool
   B. Appreciating that people do not always express pain the same way
   C. Recognizing that the communication of pain is acceptable within all cultures
   D. Understanding that the meaning of pain varies between cultures
   E. Developing an awareness of your personal values and beliefs
2. Members of a nuclear family in most cultures include:
   A. Mother
   B. Father
   C. Grandfather
   D. Grandmother
   E. Children
   F. Aunts
   G. Uncles

UNIT II

The Nursing Role in Preparing Families for Childbearing and Childrearing

CHAPTER 4

Reproductive and Sexual Health

CHAPTER OVERVIEW

Chapter 4 reviews the anatomy and physiology of the reproductive system. It addresses sexuality as it relates to each stage of growth and development in the lives of human beings. The nurse's role in providing sex education to children, adolescents, and adults is illustrated through teaching concepts in this chapter. A case study is included to provide research exposure on the current national health concerns and goals.

LEARNING OBJECTIVES

After mastering the content in this chapter, you should be able to do the following:

1. Describe anatomy and physiology necessary for reproductive and sexual health.
2. Assess a couple for anatomic and physiologic readiness for childrearing, biologic gender, gender role, and gender identity.
3. Formulate nursing diagnoses related to reproductive or sexual health.
4. Identify appropriate outcomes for reproductive and sexual health education.
5. Plan nursing care related to anatomic and physiologic readiness for childbearing or sexual health, such as helping adolescents discuss concerns in these areas.
6. Implement nursing care related to reproductive health, such as educating for menstruation.
7. Evaluate outcome criteria for achievement and effectiveness of care.
8. Identify National Health Goals related to reproductive health and sexuality and specific ways that nurses can help the nation achieve these goals.
9. Identify areas of care in relation to reproductive and sexual health that could benefit from additional nursing research or application of evidence-based practice.
10. Use critical thinking to analyze ways that clients' reproductive and sexual health can be improved for healthier childbearing and adult health.
11. Integrate knowledge of reproductive health and sexuality with the nursing process to achieve quality maternal and child health nursing care.

KEY TERMS

adrenarche
andrology
anteflexion
anteversion
aspermia
bicornuate uterus
biologic gender
culdoscopy
cystocele
dysfunction
dyspareunia
endocervix
endometrium
erectile
gender identity
gender role
gonad
gynecology
gynecomastia
heterosexual
homosexual
laparoscopy
lesbian
menarche
menopause
menorrhagia
metrorrhagia
myometrium
oocyte
perimetrium
premature ejaculation
rectocele
retroflexion
retroversion
thelarche
transsexual
transvestite
vaginismus
voyeurism

■ Mastering the Information

MATCHING

Match the terms in Column II with a definition, example, or related statement from Column I. Place the letter corresponding to the answer in the space provided.

COLUMN I

1. ____Inner sense a person has of being male or female
2. ____Ridge of tissue formed by the posterior joining of the labia minora and the labia majora
3. ____Structure located bilateral to the urinary meatus; supplies lubrication to external genitalia during coitus
4. ____Sexual fulfillment with members of the same sex
5. ____Structure contains four parts: interstitium, isthmus, ampulla, and infundibula
6. ____A pad of adipose tissue located over the symphysis pubis
7. ____Term used to denote chromosomal sexual development
8. ____Structure that serves to support and protect the reproductive and other pelvic organs
9. ____Structure that accommodates the growing fetus during pregnancy
10. ____Elastic semicircle of tissue that covers the opening of the vagina
11. ____Small, rounded organ of erectile tissue at the forward junction of the labia minora; sensitive to touch and temperature and is the center of sexual arousal

COLUMN II

a. Fallopian tubes
b. Uterus
c. Homosexual
d. Mons veneris
e. Clitoris
f. Fourchette
g. Biologic gender
h. Pelvis
i. Hymen
j. Skene's glands
k. Gender identity

TRUE OR FALSE

Indicate if the following statements are true or false by placing a "T" or "F" in the space provided.

Mrs. Bell telephones the nurse in a health care center because she would like information regarding ovulation. She states that she has a 28-day menstrual cycle and would like to know when she should expect ovulation to occur. In advising Mrs. Bell the nurse would know that:

_____1. Ovulation occurs at the midpoint of this woman's menstrual cycle.

_____2. Basal body temperature is affected by the production of progesterone and is lowered just prior to ovulation.

■ Applying Your Knowledge

CASE STUDY

As a summer student taking an independent study course, you are a mentor for a group of prospective college students. These students are matriculating in a post-high school program for persons pursuing health careers. To complete their curriculum, you must address the following principles of reproductive and sexual health:

1. State the primary role of the nurse in the promotion of reproductive health.
2. Describe four physiologic functions that explain how the activity of the hypothalamus influences the menstrual cycle.
3. Identify three environmental factors that may influence the preschooler's gender identity.
4. Summarize the physiological changes that occur in older adults that may alter the ability of both male and female to be sexually active.
5. Identify National Health Goals related to reproductive and sexual health and how the nurse may help the nation to achieve these goals.

CRITICAL INQUIRY EXERCISE

Create a teaching plan to be used in a group setting for teenage girls. Describe how conception takes place, using the sequel approach from the point of ovulation.

CRITICAL EXPLORATION

Visit a public health department and assess the approach the nurse uses to teach about reproductive health care to patients who are requesting birth control measures for the first time.

■ Practicing for NCLEX

MULTIPLE-CHOICE QUESTIONS

Circle the letter that corresponds to the best answer for each question.

1. The nurse is counseling 11-year-old Mandy and her mother in an ambulatory health care setting. The mother is communicating concerns to the nurse with regard to anticipatory guidance about menstruation. Mandy has not reached menarche. The family appears receptive and interested about the importance of health care. The nurse would know that including menstruation as a part of health education on this visit would be important because:
   A. Menopausal changes that could be a threat to Mandy's health may be occurring.
   B. Menarche should have occurred at age 9.
   C. Mandy is in jeopardy for experiencing regular cyclic hormonal changes.
   D. Menstruation is considered to be an initiation to sexuality and womanhood.

2. Some couples experience sexual dysfunction. When the female does not experience an orgasm because the male ejaculates before he desires, the dysfunction is referred to as:
   A. Dyspareunia
   B. Premature vaginismus
   C. Premature ejaculation
   D. Failure to achieve orgasm

3. A condition that causes the female to experience pain during coitus, and is usually caused by endometriosis, vaginal infection, or hormonal changes, is called:
   A. Dyspareunia
   B. Premature vaginismus
   C. Sadomasochism
   D. Fetishism

ALTERNATE FORMAT QUESTIONS

Fill in the Blank

Supply the missing term or the information requested.

1. The ——— is the body organ that produces sex cells.
2. ——— is the stage of life at which menstrual cycles cease.
3. ——— is the initiation of breast development influenced by estrogen.

Multiple-Answer Multiple Choice

Circle the letter(s) corresponding to the appropriate answer(s). Select all that apply.

1. Secretion by the seminal vesicles is high in:
   A. Sugar
   B. Protein
   C. Electrolytes
   D. Prostaglandins
   E. Acids

2. Structures associated with the female reproductive system include:
   A. Labia minora
   B. Vas deferens
   C. Ovaries
   D. Labia majora
   E. Seminal vesicles

CHAPTER 5

Reproductive Life Planning

CHAPTER OVERVIEW

Chapter 5 discusses the methods available for reproductive life planning. These methods are presented with their physiologic actions and the impact on future pregnancies. The chapter examines the process of ovulation and potential side effects of an ovulation-suppressing agent. The principles of therapeutic communication when counseling the family who seeks health care on reproductive life planning are also discussed. Case studies are provided to assist the student in learning why specific methods of reproductive life planning are recommended over other available methods.

LEARNING OBJECTIVES

After mastering the content in this chapter, you should be able to do the following:

1. Describe common methods of reproductive life planning and the advantages, disadvantages, and risk factors associated with each.
2. Assess clients for reproductive life planning needs.
3. Formulate nursing diagnoses related to reproductive life planning concerns.
4. Identify expected outcomes for couples desiring reproductive life planning.
5. Plan nursing care related to reproductive life planning, such as helping a client select a suitable family planning measure.
6. Implement nursing care related to reproductive life planning, such as educating adolescents about the use of condoms as a safer sex practice as well as preventing unwanted pregnancy.
7. Evaluate outcome criteria for achievement and effectiveness of care.
8. Identify National Health Goals related to reproductive life planning that nurses can be instrumental in helping the nation achieve.
9. Identify areas related to reproductive life planning that could benefit from additional nursing research or application of evidence-based practice.
10. Use critical thinking to analyze ways reproductive health planning can promote reproductive health within a family-centered framework.
11. Integrate reproductive life planning with the nursing process to achieve quality maternal and child health nursing care.

KEY TERMS

abstinence
barrier method
basal body temperature method
calendar method
cervical cap
coitus interruptus
condom
contraceptive
diaphragm
elective termination of pregnancy
fertility awareness
intrauterine device
laparoscopy
monophasic
natural family planning
reproductive life planning
triphasic
tubal ligation
vasectomy

■ Mastering the Information

MATCHING

Match the terms in Column II with a definition, example, or related statement from Column I. Place the letter corresponding to the answer in the space provided.

COLUMN I

1. _____Excision and blocking of the vas deferens to prevent passage of the spermatozoa
2. _____Production of antibodies against Rh-positive blood
3. _____A result of an accidental injection of saline solution into a blood vessel
4. _____Removal of the uterine lining by suction or a syringe
5. _____Contraceptive method with a 0% failure rate

COLUMN II

a. Hypernatremia
b. Menstrual extraction
c. Isoimmunization
d. Vasectomy
e. Abstinence

SHORT ANSWER

Supply the missing term or the information requested.

1. Describe three physiologic functions that suppress ovulation when "the pill" is used as a method of contraception.

2. Describe how the "minipill" differs from the traditional oral contraceptive.

3. Discuss the use of IUDs, spermicides, and condoms by adolescents as methods of reproductive life planning.

■ Applying Your Knowledge

CASE STUDY

Friday, April 20, marks 1 week since Mrs. Nugent gave birth to a 6-pound, 7.5-ounce son. She has elected to use an oral contraceptive as her reproductive life planning method after his delivery. The physician prescribes an oral contraceptive to be taken for 21 days. Mrs. Nugent tells the nurse she is not clear about when to take her pills.

1. What instructions should the nurse give Mrs. Nugent on starting the use of this oral contraceptive?

2. How often should Mrs. Nugent take the pills, and when should she expect her menstrual flow to begin?

3. What are some suggestions that the nurse can offer Mrs. Nugent to help her remember to take her pill?

Ms. Jordan brings her 16-year-old daughter Tammy to the physician's office. Tammy experienced menarche 2 months ago and Ms. Jordan suspects she is sexually active. Ms. Jordan is requesting an oral contraceptive as a method for reproductive life planning for her daughter.

1. What permanent damage may occur if use of the oral contraceptive begins before the cycle is regulated?

2. Explain the relationship between oral contraception and the potential for alteration in skeletal growth with adolescent girls.

Mrs. Patterson, age 40, married and the mother of three children, is visiting the health care center to electively terminate her pregnancy at 8 weeks of gestation. She visits the community health care facility to be counseled on the procedure. As she is being examined, she asks the nurse if terminating her pregnancy would reflect negatively on her as a patient.

1. What are some very important guidelines that the nurse must remember when responding to Mrs. Patterson?

2. Mrs. Patterson is administered a laminaria for dilation of the cervix. Why would Mrs. Patterson be routinely placed on antibiotic therapy with this procedure?

CRITICAL INQUIRY EXERCISE

1. Prepare a nursing care plan to provide health education and counseling for a patient who will be undergoing an elective tubal ligation. Focus on the future implications of the procedure.

2. Prepare a teaching plan for an adolescent who is pregnant and has expressed a desire to learn about contraceptives. The plan should address safer sex and a suitable method of reproductive life planning.

CRITICAL EXPLORATION

1. Use the teaching plan that you constructed for the above exercise to teach a teen group in a community health care setting about safer sex and reproductive life planning.

2. Survey the retail market for condoms that are self-lubricated and treated with nonoxynol-9. Present your findings when counseling the adolescent in a clinical setting.

■ Practicing for NCLEX

MULTIPLE-CHOICE QUESTIONS

Circle the letter that corresponds to the best answer for each question.

1. A procedure using carbon dioxide and the coagulation and sealing of the fallopian tubes is called:
   A. culdoscopy
   B. laparoscopy
   C. hysterectomy
   D. minilaparotomy

2. What day of the week after the start of menstrual flow should a woman begin taking an oral contraceptive?
   A. Sunday
   B. Monday
   C. Wednesday
   D. Saturday

3. When counseling an adolescent girl who expresses a desire to begin using the oral contraceptive method of reproductive life planning, it is highly recommended that the duration of her menstrual cycle be well established. How long should she have been experiencing menses before beginning to take the oral contraceptive?
   A. 1 year
   B. 2 years
   C. 3 years
   D. 4 years

4. Which of the following is thought to be a side effect of Depo-Provera?
   A. Thrombophlebitis
   B. Weight gain
   C. Excessive menstrual flow
   D. Osteoporosis

ALTERNATE FORMAT QUESTIONS

Fill in the Blank

Supply the missing term or the information requested.

1. ——— prevents pregnancy by collecting the spermatozoa before they can be deposited in the vagina.

2. A ——— is a circular rubber disk that fits over the cervix to form a barrier against the entrance of spermatozoa.

Multiple-Answer Multiple Choice

Circle the letter(s) corresponding to the appropriate answer(s). Select all that apply.

1. Identify the effects that may be associated with use of an oral contraceptive.
   A. Nausea
   B. Weight loss
   C. Headache
   D. Breast tenderness
   E. Alternating cycles

2. Select the physiological functions that suppress ovulation when the pill is used as a contraceptive. Circle all that apply.
   A. Suppression of follicle-simulating hormone
   B. Interference with progesterone secretion
   C. Increase in amount of cervical mucus
   D. Decrease in cervical mucus permeability
   E. Suppression of luteinizing hormone

CHAPTER 6

The Infertile Couple

CHAPTER OVERVIEW

Chapter 6 presents an overview of clients with fertility problems. The underlying physiologic and psychological bases for infertility problems are discussed. The use of the nursing process to address the needs of clients coping with infertility is explored.

LEARNING OBJECTIVES

After mastering the content in this chapter, you should be able to do the following:

1. Describe common causes of infertility in men and women.
2. Describe common assessments necessary to detect infertility.
3. Formulate nursing diagnoses related to infertility.
4. Identify appropriate outcomes for the infertile couple.
5. Plan interventions to meet the needs of the couple with a diagnosis of infertility.
6. Assist with interventions associated with the diagnosis of infertility or measures to promote fertility, such as health teaching.
7. Evaluate outcomes for achievement and effectiveness of care.
8. Identify National Health Goals related to infertility that nurses can participate in helping the nation achieve.
9. Identify areas of nursing care related to fertility that could benefit from additional nursing research or application of evidence-based practice.
10. Use critical thinking to analyze nursing strategies that can be used to support an infertile couple.
11. Integrate knowledge about infertility with the nursing process to achieve quality maternal and child health nursing care.

KEY TERMS

anovulation
artificial insemination
cryptorchidism
endometriosis
erectile dysfunction
in vitro fertilization
primary infertility
secondary infertility
sperm count
sperm motility infertility
spermatogenesis mumps orchitis
sterility
subfertility
varicocele

■ Mastering the Information

MATCHING

Match the terms in Column II with a definition, example, or related statement from Column I. Place the letter corresponding to the answer in the space provided.

COLUMN I

1. ____The inability to conceive a child or sustain a pregnancy to childbirth
2. ____The production of sperm cells
3. ____Introduction of a thin, hollow, lighted tube through the abdomen to examine the ovaries and uterus
4. ____A test for ovulation involving monitoring a monthly graph to determine when ovulation occurs
5. ____The inability to conceive because of a known condition
6. ____Enlargement of a testicular vein; may result in infertility due to venous congestion
7. ____Absent ova production
8. ____X-ray examination of the fallopian tubes using a radiopaque medium to evaluate tubal patency

9. ____The couple cannot conceive a child at present but has had a previous viable pregnancy.

10. ____Implantation of uterine nodules to locations outside the uterus

COLUMN II

a. Anovulation
b. Hysterosalpingography
c. Basal body temperature
d. Endometriosis
e. Infertility
f. Laparoscopy
g. Secondary infertility
h. Spermatogenesis
i. Sterility
j. Varicocele

SHORT ANSWER

Supply the missing term or the information requested.

1. Depending on a couple's motivations for fertility testing, their reaction to study results may vary from ——— to ——— ——— to ———.
2. A ——— ——— is a woman who agrees to be impregnated by a man's sperm and carry the child for him and his partner.
3. When vaginal pH is ———, sperm motility is limited or destroyed.
4. ——— ——— is the instillation of sperm into the uterus to aid conception.
5. ——— ——— fertilization involves exposing an egg to sperm outside the woman's body and transferring the embryo.

■ Applying Your Knowledge

CASE STUDY

Marilyn and Palo Jaketes have been married for 3 years. For the past year they have had unprotected sex an average of three or four times per week in an effort to conceive. They have come to the clinic for assessment and counseling.

1. How might the ages of Mr. and Mrs. Jaketes affect their fertility evaluation and possible solutions for infertility?
2. What cultural beliefs might the Jaketes have that should be considered when discussing measures to facilitate fertility? How might cultural beliefs affect their choice of alternatives to childbirth?
3. What measures could you take to support the Jaketes through their emotional responses to news of infertility?

CRITICAL INQUIRY EXERCISE

1. Prepare a teaching plan for an infertile couple that outlines various options.
2. When might adoption be an unacceptable option for a couple?

CRITICAL EXPLORATION

Explore the facilities in your city to which you might refer clients with infertility problems (e.g., sperm or egg banks, infertility clinics, and adoption agencies).

■ Practicing for NCLEX

MULTIPLE-CHOICE QUESTIONS

Circle the letter that corresponds to the best answer for each question.

1. Which of the following is true about fertility studies?
   A. Fertility studies should be undertaken more quickly with younger women.
   B. If a couple is very anxious about infertility, studies should not be delayed regardless of the couple's age.
   C. Initial testing involves primarily the partner who is suspected of being infertile.
   D. Women under 30 years of age should be referred for evaluation after 6 months of infertility.

2. Diane has been told she has blocked fallopian tubes. Which of the following fertility options should the nurse help her to explore?
   A. Hormonal therapy
   B. Artificial insemination
   C. In vitro fertilization
   D. Gamete intrafallopian transfer

3. Which of the following suggestions would be most appropriate to give to a couple to aid conception?
   A. Having coitus every day will increase chances for fertility.
   B. Douching should be done before coitus to promote sperm mobility.
   C. The male-superior position for coitus is best to achieve conception by placing sperm near the cervix.
   D. The woman should ambulate immediately after coitus to mobilize the egg toward sperm.

ALTERNATE FORMAT QUESTIONS

Fill in the Blank

Supply the missing term or the information requested.

1. A uterine endometrial ——— may result in symptoms of bleeding and clot passage after the procedure.

2. A woman who is allergic to iodine and is scheduled for a hysterosalpingogram is considered to at risk for an ——————— reaction .

Multiple-Answer Multiple Choice

Circle the letter(s) corresponding to the appropriate answer(s). Select all that apply.

1. What measures may be appropriate for a man to take to increase his sperm count?
   A. Increase frequency of coitus.
   B. Wear clothing that does not restrict or overheat the scrotum.
   C. Avoid frequent use of hot baths.
   D. Increase alcohol intake.
   E. Increase sport activities.

2. When discussing the benefits associated with childless living with a couple who is infertile, which of the following would the nurse include?
   A. Career growth
   B. Pursuit of hobbies
   C. Antisocial behaviors
   D. Personal contributions to society
   E. Continuance of education

UNIT III

The Nursing Role in Caring for the Pregnant Family

CHAPTER 7

Genetic Assessment and Counseling

CHAPTER OVERVIEW

Chapter 7 presents an overview of basic principles and concepts related to genetic assessment and counseling. The inheritance of disease and types of genetic defects are discussed. The role of nurses in genetic counseling and the care of clients with genetic disorders is explored.

LEARNING OBJECTIVES

After mastering the content in this chapter, you should be able to do the following:

1. Describe the nature of inheritance and patterns of recessive and dominant mendelian inheritance and common chromosomal aberrations, such as nondisjunction syndromes.
2. Assess a family for the probability of inheriting a genetic disorder.
3. Formulate nursing diagnoses related to genetic disorders.
4. Establish outcomes that meet the needs of the pregnant family undergoing genetic assessment and counseling.
5. Plan nursing care related to an alteration in genetic health, such as assisting with an amniocentesis.
6. Implement nursing care related to identification of or counseling for a genetic disorder.
7. Evaluate outcomes for achievement and effectiveness of nursing care.
8. Identify National Health Goals and specific measures related to genetic disorders that nurses can take to help the nation achieve these goals.
9. Identify areas related to genetic assessment that could benefit from additional nursing research.
10. Use critical thinking to analyze ways that nurses can contribute to health education and counseling for genetic issues.
11. Integrate knowledge of genetic inheritance with the nursing process to achieve quality maternal and child health nursing care.

KEY TERMS

alleles
chromosomes
dermatoglyphics
dominant
genes
genetics
genome
genotype
heterozygous trait
homozygous trait
imprinting
karyotype
meiosis
nondisjunction
phenotype
recessive gene

■ Mastering the Information

MATCHING

Match the terms in Column II with a definition, example, or related statement from Column I. Place the letter corresponding to the answer in the space provided.

COLUMN I

1. _____Expression of genetic material allowing identification of whether chromosomal material has come from the male or female parent
2. _____Specific point on a chromosome marking the location of a missing or abnormal gene
3. _____A woman agreeing to undergo artificial insemination by the male partner's sperm and to bear a child for the couple
4. _____Material of heredity, strands of genes in the nucleus of body cells
5. _____When paired with other genes, these genes always be expressed.
6. _____Ability to be passed from one generation to the next
7. _____Visual inspection of the chromosome pattern
8. _____Having two like genes for a trait
9. _____An outward appearance or expression of the genes

COLUMN II

a. Genetic disorder
b. Chromosomes
c. Phenotype
d. Imprinting
e. Homozygous
f. Surrogate
g. Dominant gene
h. Genetic marker
i. Karyotyping

SHORT ANSWER

Supply the missing term or the information requested.

1. Discuss the merits of genetic testing for a couple at risk for having a child with an incurable genetic disease.

2. Differentiate between the chance of inheriting a disease if both parents are heterozygous for the trait and the disease is dominantly inherited, and the chance of inheritance if the disease is recessively inherited.

3. Discuss two of the four main purposes of genetic counseling.

4. Discuss why genetic counseling might be ineffective after the diagnosis of the pregnancy or immediately after the birth of a child with a defect.

■ Applying Your Knowledge

CASE STUDY

Bell and Bennie Johnson, both 32 years old, have been married for 1 year and want to have a baby. Bell has come for a complete physical and states she's concerned that she is too old for a healthy pregnancy. While doing the history, the nurse discovers Bell has a brother with Duchenne muscular dystrophy (DMD).

1. What is the significance of X-linked inheritance in determining the chances that Bell will have a baby with DMD if Bell is a carrier?

2. If Bell gives birth to a child with DMD, what nursing actions would be appropriate to help Bennie and Bell in planning for the future needs of their family and the child? Would it be appropriate for the nurse to approach family members, explain the genetic defect, and encourage them to support the couple? Why or why not?

CRITICAL INQUIRY EXERCISE

1. Write a brief statement on your opinion regarding the use of amniocentesis to determine if a fetus is without defects and if the couple should continue or terminate the pregnancy.

2. How might testing to determine the gender of an infant become an ethical dilemma? What are your thoughts regarding the use of modern technology to determine the gender of a child when a gender-specific genetic disorder is possible? When no disorder is likely?

CRITICAL EXPLORATION

Attend a genetic counseling session and write a short report on the content discussed and reactions noted from the couple.

■ Practicing for NCLEX

MULTIPLE-CHOICE QUESTIONS

Circle the letter that corresponds to the best answer for each question.

1. If "large feet" is a recessive trait and one parent is heterozygous for the trait and the other parent is homozygous for the trait, what are the chances that a child of this union will have large feet?
   A. 25% (1 in 4)
   B. 50% (2 in 4)
   C. 75% (3 in 4)
   D. 100% (4 in 4)

2. Which of the following individuals must be heterozygous for the recessive disease trait?
   A. Adam, who has no symptoms of the disease but has passed it on to his child
   B. Barbara, who displays no symptoms and has no children with the disease
   C. Peter, who has symptoms of the disease and has an affected child
   D. Wendy, who has symptoms of the disease but has no affected child

3. Which of the following couples would benefit most from referral for immediate genetic counseling?
   A. Tom, age 50, and Alice, age 42, who have just discovered they are going to have a baby
   B. Jim and Melissa, who have just had an infant with cystic fibrosis
   C. John and Jean, who want to have a baby but only want a male child
   D. Pete, who has hemophilia, and DeeDee, who have been married for a year and want to have a child

4. What role would be most appropriate for the nurse involved with genetic counseling?
   A. Assess the options available to a couple and select the best ones to present for the couple to choose from
   B. Inform the couple of the procedures they may undergo in genetic screening and in genetic counseling.
   C. Instruct parents on the need for an immediate abortion if both persons have the trait for a dominant disease.
   D. Limit the information provided to the couple about the genetic defect to avoid influencing their decision.

5. To determine if a disorder occurred by chance or is carried by family members, a nurse should collect which of the following data?
   A. A history of the couple's sexual pattern during the time of conception
   B. As complete a family history of infant deaths or abnormalities as possible
   C. A prenatal history of nausea and reports of back pain in the last trimester
   D. Physical assessment of the infant's eye and hair color

6. Nursing measures that may be implemented when preparing a woman for amniocentesis should include which of the following?
   A. Determining that the woman is in her fifth to eighth week of pregnancy
   B. Discussing the 10% risk that premature labor will be stimulated
   C. Supporting the woman who is beginning to accept the pregnancy and bond with the fetus
   D. Explaining that the procedure involves scanning with no invasive measures

ALTERNATE FORMAT QUESTIONS

Fill in the Blank

Supply the missing term or the information requested.

1. Health professionals have a legal and ________ obligation to share genetic information with the involved couple and no one else.
2. Genetic counseling will inform a couple about the genetic disorder and the chances that their child might ________________________ it.

Multiple-Answer Multiple Choice

Circle the letter(s) corresponding to the appropriate answer(s). Select all that apply.

1. Couples who undergo genetic counseling and are informed that they have a genetic abnormality in the family and might have a child with a genetic defect may experience which of the following behaviors?
   A. Loss of self-esteem
   B. Blame
   C. Embarrassment
   D. Joy
   E. Anger
   F. Depression

2. Which of the following would be appropriate guidance to give a couple found to be at high risk for producing a child with an inherited disease or defect?
   A. Delivery through cesarean section instead of vaginal delivery
   B. Implantation of a donor embryo if the female has the inherited trait
   C. Repair of fetal defects outside the uterus after fertilization
   D. Using the Lamaze method, which would reduce the risk of defects
   E. Hemophilia is an illness that can be inherited.

CHAPTER 8

The Growing Fetus

CHAPTER OVERVIEW

The development of the fetus is a complex phenomenon that originates from the union of an ovum and a sperm. When united, the ovum and the sperm form a single cell called the zygote. This chapter allows the student to explore all the stages of fetal development, enabling him or her to help the childbearing family understand the changes that take place during pregnancy. The student is also challenged to learn nursing principles necessary to conduct fetal monitoring and convey findings to the members of the childbearing family.

LEARNING OBJECTIVES

After mastering the content in this chapter, you should be able to do the following:

1. Describe the growth and development of the fetus by gestation week.
2. Assess fetal growth and development through maternal and pregnancy landmarks.
3. Formulate nursing diagnoses related to the needs of the pregnant woman and developing fetus.
4. Establish outcome criteria that meet the needs of the growing fetus.
5. Plan nursing care that promotes healthy fetal growth.
6. Implement nursing care to help ensure a safe pregnancy outcome and a safe fetal environment.
7. Evaluate expected outcomes for achievement and effectiveness of care.
8. Identify National Health Goals related to fetal growth that nurses can help the nation to achieve.
9. Identify areas of fetal health that could benefit from additional nursing research or application of evidence-based practice.
10. Use critical thinking to analyze ways to promote fetal growth and development and make care family-centered, even at this early point in life.
11. Integrate knowledge of fetal growth and development with the nursing process to achieve quality maternal and child health nursing care.

KEY TERMS

amniocentesis
amniotic cavity
amniotic membrane
blastocyst
cephalocaudal
chorionic membrane
chorionic villi
cotyledons
ductus arteriosus
ductus venosus
embryo
entoderm
expected date of birth
fertilization
fetoscopy
fetus
foramen ovale
hydramnios
implantation
lightening
McDonald's rule
morula
neural plate
nonstress test
oligohydramnios
organogenesis
quickening
surfactant
trophoblast
umbilical cord
yolk sac
zygote

■ Mastering the Information

MATCHING

Match the terms in Column II with a definition, example, or related statement from Column I. Place the letter corresponding to the answer in the space provided.

COLUMN I

1. ____ Three-part organ (basalis, capsularis, and vera) that is discarded following the birth of a child
2. ____ Hormone found in the bloodstream shortly after conception and prior to first missed menstrual period

3. ____Transvaginal aspiration of fluid that collects in the extraembryonic cavity in early pregnancy
4. ____Aspiration of amniotic fluid from the pregnant uterus for examination
5. ____A method of determining that the fetus is growing in utero by measuring fundal (uterine) height
6. ____A developmental pattern that proceeds from head to tail
7. ____Contact between the blastocyst and the uterine endothelium occurring approximately 8 to 10 days after fertilization
8. ____A gelatinous mucopolysaccharide that gives the umbilical cord body and prevents pressure on the vein and arteries
9. ____Important function in transporting oxygen and nutrients to the fetus from the placenta and returning waste products from the fetus to the placenta
10. ____A phospholipid substance that decreases alveolar surface tension on expiration

COLUMN II

a. Implantation
b. Amniocentesis
c. Surfactant
d. Decidua
e. Umbilical cord
f. McDonald's rule
g. Wharton's jelly
h. Human chorionic gonadotropin
i. Cephalocaudal
j. Coelocentesis

CHRONOLOGICAL ORDER

Assign the correct gestational age to the description and place in order from the beginning to the end of fetal life.

Week of Gestation	*Description of Fetus*
______	Heart has septum and valves. Facial features are definitely discernible.
______	Average weight is 1,600 g; assumes delivery position; stores iron.
______	Additional deposits of subcutaneous fat and lanugo start to diminish.
______	Average weight is 1,200 g; lung alveoli begin maturing with surfactant.
______	Formation of lanugo; liver and pancreas are functioning; fetus demonstrates swallowing reflex.
______	Quickening experienced by the mother; beginning of vernix caseosa
______	Nail beds forming on toes and fingers; tooth buds present; heart sounds audible by Doppler instrument
______	Average weight is 550 g; passive antibody transfer from mother to fetus.

SHORT ANSWER

Explain how nutrients are exchanged from the mother to the fetus during pregnancy.

■ Applying Your Knowledge

CASE STUDY

Mrs. Menendez is 44 years of age and at 28 weeks' gestation. She is admitted to the hospital after experiencing acute abdominal pain for several days. The physician orders a biophysical profile procedure to determine the well-being of the fetus.

1. How many parameters are to be considered in the biophysical profile?
2. What is the highest potential score for each parameter?
3. Explain the reliability of the biophysical profile as an assessment tool.
4. How are the assessment findings used to determine the criteria score?
5. What major roles does the nurse play in obtaining the information for a biophysical profile?

CRITICAL INQUIRY EXERCISE

1. Construct a diagram to illustrate how a couple may use the woman's body metabolic temperature as an indicator to predict ovulation. Demonstrate how coitus occurring 1 to 2 days before ovulation, as well as after ovulation, can result in fertilization.

2. Use colorful markers to draw a diagram of fetal circulation. Ask your instructor to allot you a portion of your laboratory class time to present your diagram. Name all anatomical structures of fetal circulation and discuss their functions.

CRITICAL EXPLORATION

Formulate a nursing care plan expected outcome that addresses adequate fetal oxygenation throughout gestation. Then visit a health clinic on a day that several prenatal patients are scheduled to be seen. Note all of the implementations and procedures of the health care provider that can be viewed as actions to accomplish your goal.

■ Practicing for NCLEX

MULTIPLE-CHOICE QUESTIONS

Circle the letter that corresponds to the best answer for each question.

1. Beverly is being seen on her first prenatal visit at the health care clinic in her community. She reports that the first day of her last menstrual period was May 7, 2007. As calculated by Nagele's rule, Beverly's EDC will be:
   A. New Year's Day 2008 (1-1-08)
   B. Valentine's Day 2008 (2-14-08)
   C. Veterans Day 2008 (11-12-08)
   D. April Fool's Day 2008 (4-1-08)

2. Mr. and Mrs. Mitchell are expecting their first child. On their visit to the physician's office for a scheduled appointment, they are jubilant over the pregnancy and curious about the health care procedures. As the nurse prepares Mrs. Mitchell for her assessment, she uses the Doppler to listen for the fetal heart tone. The nurse will expect the heart tone to be in a normal range of:
   A. 110 to 120
   B. 120 to 160
   C. 170 to 180
   D. 180 to 200

3. The nurse is preparing Mrs. Mitchell for an ultrasound. Which action would be most appropriate?
   A. Instruct her to empty her bladder.
   B. Have her drink 8 ounces of water every 15 minutes for 90 minutes before the procedure.
   C. Shave her abdomen.
   D. Place Mrs. Mitchell in semi-Fowler's position with legs elevated.

4. Mr. Mitchell asks the nurse to explain why his wife needs an ultrasound. The nurse would respond appropriately by stating:
   A. "An ultrasound is a common examination to monitor how the infant is growing and moving and to check for any complications."
   B. "The ultrasound test is used to measure the length and weight of your baby and to detect any chromosome abnormalities."
   C. "The ultrasound test is given to every pregnant woman. The explanation for why the test is given is complicated, but we will certainly let you know if the results are abnormal."
   D. "The doctor will explain the test to you, but I can tell you that we are checking to see if there are any problems with the pregnancy."

5. Mrs. Morrell complained of discomfort after having had an amniocentesis procedure. She is at 20 weeks' gestation and is 45 years old. Which of the following symptoms would prompt immediate action?
   A. Lab results reveal abnormal chromosome cells.
   B. Amniotic fluid contains fetal urine.
   C. Mrs. Morrell reports moderate vaginal bleeding.
   D. Mrs. Morrell describes symptoms of Braxton Hicks contractions.

ALTERNATE FORMAT QUESTIONS

Fill in the Blank

Supply the missing term or the information requested.

1. The second fetal membrane lining the chorionic membrane is the ———— ———— membrane.
2. ——— occurs when the fetus is unable to swallow.

Multiple-Answer Multiple Choice

Circle the letter(s) corresponding to the appropriate answer(s). Select all that apply.

1. Which of the following structures are derived from the ectoderm germ layer?
   A. Sebaceous glands
   B. Brain
   C. Bladder
   D. Heart
   E. Skin
   F. Sense organs

2. The nurse would explain which of the following when teaching a pregnant woman about the information obtained with a biophysical profile?
   A. Fetal breathing
   B. Fetal movement
   C. Fetal tone
   D. Amniotic fluid volume
   E. Fetal heart rate reactivity
   F. Lecithin/sphingomyelin ratio

CHAPTER 9

Psychological and Physiologic Changes of Pregnancy

CHAPTER OVERVIEW

Chapter 9 addresses the psychological and physical changes a woman and her partner undergo during pregnancy. Though the physiologic changes of pregnancy are dynamic and extensive, they are considered an extension of normal physiology. The nurse uses this concept when preparing teaching plans and developing care plans. At the completion of this chapter the student will be knowledgeable about the interplay of these changes. This will enable the student to understand how to promote pregnancy as an extension of wellness in the family and throughout the pregnancy and early parenthood.

LEARNING OBJECTIVES

After mastering the content in this chapter, you should be able to do the following:

1. Describe common psychological and physiologic changes that occur with pregnancy, the underlying principles for these changes, and the relationship of the changes to pregnancy diagnosis.
2. Assess a woman for the psychological and physical changes that occur with pregnancy through health history and physical examination.
3. Formulate nursing diagnoses related to the psychological and physical changes of pregnancy.
4. Identify outcome criteria for the family's psychological and physical adaptation to pregnancy.
5. Plan nursing care related to the changes and diagnosis of pregnancy, such as helping women plan to get adequate rest.
6. Implement nursing care, such as health teaching related to the expected changes of pregnancy.
7. Evaluate outcome criteria for the achievement and effectiveness of care.
8. Identify National Health Goals that nurses could be instrumental in helping the nation achieve.
9. Identify areas of nursing care related to the psychological and physiologic changes of pregnancy that could benefit from additional nursing research.
10. Use critical thinking to analyze how the physical and psychological changes of pregnancy affect family functioning, and develop ways to make nursing care more family-centered.
11. Integrate knowledge of the psychological and physiologic changes in pregnancy with the nursing process to achieve quality maternal and child health nursing care.

KEY TERMS

ballottement
Braxton Hicks contractions
Chadwick's sign
couvade syndrome
diastasis
Goodell's sign
Hegar's sign
hyperptyalism
lightening
melasma
Montgomery's tubercles
multipara
operculum
polyuria
positive signs of pregnancy
presumptive signs of pregnancy
primigravida
probable signs of pregnancy
pseudoanemia
striae gravidarum

■ Mastering The Information

MATCHING

Match the terms in Column II with the signs of pregnancy listed in Column I. Place the letter corresponding to the answer in the space provided.

COLUMN I

1. ____Positive test for hCG hormone in urine
2. ____Palpation of fetal movements

3. ____Quickening
4. ____Chadwick's sign
5. ____Striae gravidarum
6. ____Auscultation of fetal heart sounds
7. ____Fetal outline felt by examiner
8. ____Breast changes
9. ____Braxton Hicks contractions
10. ____Sonographic fetal gestational sac
11. ____Ballottement

COLUMN II

a. Presumptive sign of pregnancy
b. Probable sign of pregnancy
c. Positive sign of pregnancy

SHORT ANSWER

Supply the missing term or the information requested.

1. What can the nurse do to help achieve the National Health Goals for women during pregnancy?

2. You are caring for a pregnant client in the third trimester. What is one reason why you would advise her to lie in the lateral recumbent position while sleeping?

3. What explanation would the nurse give to an expectant mother who has glucose in her urine but has tested negative for gestational diabetes?

4. Explain why it is important that pregnancy be diagnosed as early as possible and how this diagnosis may affect the woman's lifestyle and health status.

■ Applying Your Knowledge

CASE STUDY

Dove Whitewater, age 44, has come to the clinic for a pregnancy test. She is alone, appears very anxious, and has an obvious swelling around her abdominal area. She states she has been nauseated for the past 5 months and usually eats only a light lunch since food makes her sick in the morning and at night.

1. What emotions might Dove reveal when her pregnancy is confirmed?

2. What are some taboos, or prescriptive and restrictive beliefs, held by some American Indians that would be physically harmless if followed by Dove during her pregnancy?

3. Dove states she might decide to terminate her pregnancy. What would your response be?

CRITICAL INQUIRY EXERCISE

1. Develop a teaching plan that would give anticipatory guidance with reference to the acceptance of pregnancy. How might this plan be different for a single woman than for a married woman?

2. Explain how some psychological changes of pregnancy can be caused or aggravated by the physiologic changes of pregnancy.

CRITICAL EXPLORATION

1. Perform assessments on three pregnant women in the first, second, and third trimesters. Record findings from your interviews that describe the psychological tasks of accepting the pregnancy, accepting the baby, and preparing for parenthood.

2. Assess a client in the second trimester of pregnancy who is experiencing Braxton Hicks contractions. Explain the differences between these and labor contractions.

■ Practicing for NCLEX

MULTIPLE-CHOICE QUESTIONS

Circle the letter that corresponds to the best answer for each question.

1. Helga, age 21, is pregnant with her first child. She is in her second trimester and complains of problems with drooling. You would explain that:
   A. She should be admitted to the hospital to assess the cause of this unusual symptom.
   B. This symptom shows a deficiency of sodium and indicates she should increase her salt intake.
   C. Drooling is the body's way of eliminating excess fluid to prevent high blood pressure.
   D. The drooling is called "hyperptyalism" and is due to her increased hormone levels.

2. John, age 33, has just found out his girlfriend Ceilie is 4 months pregnant. Which of the following might indicate that a teaching plan is needed?
   A. John has not expressed pleasure or displeasure regarding the pregnancy.
   B. John refers to the fetus as "it" when talking to Ceilie about the pregnancy.
   C. John expresses great concern that if Ceilie breastfeeds she will ruin her figure.
   D. John says he hopes Ceilie will exercise more so she might have an easy vaginal delivery.

3. Which of the following most accurately reflects the psychological tasks associated with pregnancy?
   A. During the first trimester women begin "nest-building" activities.
   B. In the second trimester women experience "quickening," which contributes to acceptance of the baby.
   C. During the third trimester the father-to-be usually begins the process of accepting the pregnancy.
   D. During the first trimester the father-to-be begins preparing for parenthood.

4. Which of the following is a positive example of reworking developmental tasks?
   A. The father-to-be begins to fantasize about being a carefree bachelor.
   B. An adolescent mother-to-be states she understands why her mother made her come home before dark.
   C. The father-to-be states his partner doesn't care for him since her pregnancy.
   D. A 42-year-old mother-to-be role-plays life before pregnancy.

5. Which of the following might indicate a problem in adjustment to pregnancy?
   A. A pregnant woman whose mother was abusive to her refuses to think about or discuss it.
   B. The pregnant woman reports an increase in sexual desire and greater enjoyment of sex.
   C. The father-to-be reports that his pregnant wife has frequent mood swings.
   D. The pregnant woman shows difficulty making decisions at work and at home.

ALTERNATE FORMAT QUESTIONS

Fill in the Blank

Supply the missing term or the information requested.

1. __________ is a term used to describe the woman who has had more than one birth.
2. __________ describes a woman in her first pregnancy.

Multiple-Answer Multiple Choice

Circle the letter(s) corresponding to the appropriate answer(s). Select all that apply.

1. Which of the following changes in the gastrointestinal system are associated with pregnancy?
   A. Displacement of the stomach and intestines
   B. Constipation and flatulence
   C. Increased appetite
   D. Hyperptyalism
   E. Diarrhea

2. Which of the following are changes in the endocrine system as a result of pregnancy?
   A. Formulation of the placenta as an endocrine gland
   B. An increase in the parathyroid's size
   C. Decrease in thyroid hormone production
   D. Decrease in thyroid gland size
   E. Production of oxytocin and prolactin by the pituitary gland

CHAPTER 10

Assessing Fetal and Maternal Health: The First Prenatal Visit

CHAPTER OVERVIEW

When a woman visits a health care facility for the first prenatal visit, an assertive effort should be made by the health care providers to validate the pregnancy, determine the woman's health status and risk for complications, and initiate strategies that will encourage the woman and her family to establish positive behavior patterns of health promotion during the pregnancy and throughout their lives. This chapter allows the student to review the anatomic structures of the female body and demonstrate knowledge of how to appropriately intervene to provide nursing care, education, and guidance during the mother's pregnancy. A case study is included to help the student integrate therapeutic communication skills and nursing actions when assisting the patient with a pelvic examination.

LEARNING OBJECTIVES

After mastering the content in this chapter, you should be able to do the following:

1. Describe the areas of health assessment commonly included in a first prenatal visit.
2. Assess a pregnant woman's health status.
3. Formulate nursing diagnoses related to the health status of pregnancy.
4. Identify outcomes for achieving a healthy pregnancy.
5. Plan nursing care, such as preparing a woman for a pelvic examination or fundal measurement.
6. Implement nursing care, such as establishing a risk score for pregnancy.
7. Evaluate expected outcomes related to fetal or maternal health for achievement and effectiveness of care.
8. Identify National Health Goals that nurses can be instrumental in helping the nation to achieve.
9. Identify areas of prenatal care that could benefit from additional nursing research.
10. Use critical thinking to analyze ways to ensure family-centered prenatal care.
11. Integrate knowledge of pregnancy health assessment with the nursing process to achieve quality maternal and child health care.

KEY TERMS

abortion
age of viability
chloasma
conjugate vera
diagonal conjugate
erosion
gravida
ischial tuberosity
lithotomy position
multigravida
multipara
nulligravida
paragravida
primigravida
primipara
speculum
true conjugate

■ Mastering The Information

MATCHING

Match the anatomical areas to be examined in Column I with the correct technique from Column II. Place the letter corresponding to the answer in the space provided.

COLUMN I

1. _____ Endocervical
2. _____ Cervical os
3. _____ Posterior vaginal fornix

COLUMN II

a. Place applicator just below the cervix, rolling gently to obtain secretions. Place on laboratory slide.
b. Use a wet saline applicator and insert it through the speculum into the os of the cervix. Rotate clockwise and counterclockwise. Place on laboratory slide.

c. Press uneven end of supplied spatula on the os, rotate, and scrape cells in a circular motion. Place on laboratory slide.

TRUE OR FALSE

Indicate if the following statements are true or false by placing a "T" or "F" in the space provided.

_____ 1. The cervical os is observed as round and small in a nulligravida client.

_____ 2. Petroleum lubricant should be used on the speculum when viewing the cervix.

_____ 3. When a client has a Chlamydia infection, the vaginal mucosa appears extremely inflamed, with a greenish-yellow discharge.

_____ 4. A platypelloid pelvis accommodates childbirth with fewer difficulties than the other three types of pelves.

_____ 5. The purpose of a prenatal visit is to establish a baseline of present health and minimize the risk of possible complications.

■ Applying Your Knowledge

CASE STUDY

Mrs. Goldstein is scheduled in the prenatal clinic for a pelvic examination. She will need to be prepared for the examination of several internal and external reproductive organs.

1. What position should Mrs. Goldstein assume once she is on the examination table?

2. Name the instruments that the nurse should have available for the examination.

3. How may a support person be of assistance to Mrs. Goldstein?

4. If she is found to be positive for the HIV virus, what decisions might she need to consider?

CRITICAL INQUIRY EXERCISE

1. Diagram the four types of pelves on a poster. Illustrate to your class how the anatomy of the pelvis may accommodate or hamper the fetus as it progresses through the birthing process.

2. Determine four assessment criteria that could help determine that a pregnant woman is at high risk for HIV infection.

CRITICAL EXPLORATION

Visit a prenatal health care setting and select a patient in the third trimester of pregnancy who has been counseled and diagnosed as having a pelvis incompetent for delivery. Use your diagram as a tool to help the family understand the information discussed during counseling concerning the structure of the expectant mother's pelvis.

■ Practicing for NCLEX

MULTIPLE-CHOICE QUESTIONS

Circle the letter that corresponds to the best answer for each question.

1. A pregnant client has delayed her first prenatal visit, coming to the clinic only after she starts to experience edema of the feet and hands. The nurse takes a history and performs a physical examination. The client's response to one of the nurse's questions is, "This is my third pregnancy. I miscarried twice, the first time when I was 8 weeks pregnant and the last time when I was 26 weeks." The nurse correctly records Mrs. Barton's pregnancy status as:
   A. Gravida 2 P0
   B. Gravida 2 P1
   C. Gravida 3 P1
   D. Gravida 3 P0

2. While lying in the lithotomy position during an examination, a pregnant client complains of dizziness and nausea. What would be an appropriate nursing action to relieve the client's discomfort?
   A. Administering an antiemetic ordered by the physician
   B. Offering small sips of ginger ale
   C. Assisting the client to a side-lying position temporarily
   D. Discontinuing the examination

3. Diplopia was noted during the assessment of a pregnant client. This condition is described as:
   A. Elevated pigmentation of the skin
   B. Double vision
   C. Facial edema
   D. Gingivitis

4. Which of the following injectable vaccines would be safe to administer to a pregnant client?
   A. Varicella
   B. Measles
   C. Mumps
   D. Polio

5. A pregnant client is in her 33rd week of gestation. The nurse would assist the client in scheduling her next appointment in:
   A. 1 month
   B. 3 weeks
   C. 2 weeks
   D. 1 week

ALTERNATE FORMAT QUESTIONS

Fill in the Blank

Supply the missing term or the information requested.

1. A(n) ——— pelvis has a well-rounded inlet and a wide pubic arch.
2. In a(n) ——— pelvis, the transverse diameter is narrow and anteroposterior diameter of the inlet is larger than normal.
3. A(n) ——— pelvis has an oval-shaped inlet and is smoothly curved.
4. In a(n) ——— pelvis, the pubic arch forms an acute angle, narrowing lower dimensions of the pelvis.

Multiple-Answer Multiple Choice

Circle the letter(s) corresponding to the appropriate answer(s). Select all that apply.

1. Prior to becoming pregnant, a client was receiving the following medications. Which of these medications would be considered detrimental to the fetus during pregnancy?
   A. Acetaminophen
   B. Accutane
   C. Penicillin
   D. Folic acid
   E. Live vaccines

CHAPTER 11

Promoting Fetal and Maternal Health

CHAPTER OVERVIEW

Chapter 11 provides an overview of nursing care related to health promotion during pregnancy and the prevention of fetal exposure to teratogens. The general self-care needs of the pregnant woman, as well as common discomforts encountered during pregnancy, are reviewed. The use of the nursing process to plan and provide appropriate teaching for the woman throughout pregnancy is explored.

LEARNING OBJECTIVES

After mastering the content in this chapter, you should be able to do the following:

1. Describe health practices important for a positive pregnancy outcome.
2. Assess a woman's health practices and concerns during pregnancy.
3. Formulate nursing diagnoses to promote a healthy pregnancy.
4. Identify expected outcomes of a healthy pregnancy.
5. Plan health promotion strategies to limit exposure to teratogens or reduce the minor discomforts of pregnancy.
6. Implement care to promote positive health practices during pregnancy.
7. Evaluate expected outcomes for achievement and effectiveness of health promotion.
8. Identify National Health Goals related to pregnancy care that nurses can help the nation to achieve.
9. Identify areas of prenatal care that could benefit from additional nursing research and the application of evidence-based practice.
10. Use critical thinking to analyze ways to promote individualized and family-centered prenatal care.
11. Integrate knowledge of health promotion strategies with the nursing process to achieve quality maternal and child nursing care.

KEY TERMS

Braxton Hicks contractions
cytomegalovirus
fetal alcohol syndrome
leukorrhea
organogenesis period
Sims' position
teratogen
teratogenicity
toxoplasmosis

■ Mastering the Information

MATCHING

Match the terms in Column I with a definition, example, or related statement from Column II. Place the letter corresponding to the answer in the space provided.

COLUMN I

1. ____Braxton Hicks contractions
2. ____Cytomegalovirus
3. ____Fetal alcohol syndrome
4. ____Leukorrhea
5. ____Palmar erythema
6. ____Headache
7. ____Pelvic radiation
8. ____Modified Sims' position
9. ____Teratogen
10. ____Toxoplasmosis

COLUMN II

a. Whitish, viscous vaginal discharge
b. A possible result of expanding blood volume that puts pressure on cerebral arteries
c. Any factor, chemical or physical, that adversely affects the fertilized ovum, the embryo, or the fetus
d. A protozoan infection spread through contact with cat stool
e. Laterally lying with the abdomen on the bed and the top leg forward

f. A member of the herpes family that can cause extensive fetal damage
g. Infant who is small for gestational age, with mental retardation and characteristic craniofacial deformity
h. Symptom occurring in early pregnancy, probably caused by increased estrogen levels
i. Uterine cramps that may begin at the 8th to 12th week of pregnancy
j. Must be avoided by all women of child-bearing age except during the first 10 days of the menstrual cycle

SHORT ANSWER

Supply the missing term or the information requested.

1. What major intervention is associated with health promotion during pregnancy?
2. For each of the following activities, discuss one concept that should be discussed with the pregnant woman: bathing, breast care, perineal hygiene, dressing, sexual activity, exercise, sleep, and travel.
3. Describe five categories of potentially teratogenic drugs.
4. Discuss two instructions the nurse should provide to a pregnant woman who will be working related to all jobs, jobs requiring standing or walking, and jobs that require physical exertion.
5. Discuss how maternal stress may have a teratogenic effect.

■ Applying Your Knowledge

CASE STUDY

Ginene Varez, 31 years of age, visits your clinic for her first prenatal check-up. She is in her first trimester of pregnancy. She complains of skipping heartbeats, headache, and nausea, and states she is worried that the "tension" of her job as an accountant in a perfume factory will have a negative effect on her baby. Her blood pressure and pulse are in the normal range.

1. What would you explain to Ginene about a common physical change of pregnancy that has likely resulted in both the headache and heart palpitations?
2. What measures would you suggest to help Ginene reduce anxiety from her job?
3. If you prepared a teaching plan to help Ginene avoid teratogens, what assessments would you need to make regarding her treatment of the nausea she experiences, and her job environment?

CRITICAL INQUIRY EXERCISE

1. Prepare a teaching plan for a working woman that addresses methods for maintaining adequate nutrition and rest.
2. What are some realistic ways a pregnant woman can minimize exposure to common teratogens in the environment?

CRITICAL EXPLORATION

Observe the initial prenatal visit for women in each of the following age groups: 12 to 17, 25 to 30, and 35 to 40. Note the differences and similarities in instructions given regarding activities and rest, and nutritional needs.

■ Practicing for NCLEX

MULTIPLE-CHOICE QUESTIONS

Circle the letter that corresponds to the best answer for each question.

1. Bobby has been experiencing severe constipation during her eighth month of pregnancy. An appropriate goal or outcome criterion for Bobby would be to:
   A. Become accustomed to the constipation and accept it as unavoidable.
   B. Consume a diet containing high amounts of fiber and fruit and extra amounts of fluid.
   C. Have a bowel movement every other day to avoid daily straining activity.
   D. Refrain from taking her iron supplement, since it probably caused the problem.

2. When planning a teaching strategy for a pregnant woman, the nurse should do which of the following?
   A. Give information about how the woman can manage the specific problems she identifies as relevant in her life.
   B. Omit information related to minor pains of pregnancy to prevent the woman from developing hypochondria.
   C. Provide all information to the woman in a group session with other pregnant women so she can have someone to discuss it with.
   D. During the first prenatal visit, teach a woman the care measures necessary for health promotion throughout the pregnancy.

3. Bonnie, 6 months pregnant, is commuting 2 to 3 hours by car to school for a 6-week session. The nurse should discuss which of the following with Bonnie about travel?
   A. Dangers related to wearing lap seatbelts during the early months of pregnancy
   B. Methods of relieving stiffness and muscle aches and improving circulation during the drive
   C. The importance of taking motion sickness medications to lessen the nausea from driving
   D. The need to call her doctor and drive home immediately if she experiences premature labor or any danger signs of pregnancy

4. Sheila, 7 months pregnant, reports feeling her heart skipping a beat sometimes. The nurse recognizes these as heart palpitations and sets which of the following goal criteria? Sheila will:
   A. Demonstrate moving slowly from one position to another
   B. Lie supine when sleeping to keep pressure on her vena cava
   C. Plan a menu that includes high vitamin C content
   D. Verbalize intent to limit fluids to lower her heart's workload

5. Dee is in her second month of pregnancy and complains of abdominal pain. Which action by the nurse would be most appropriate?
   A. Encourage Dee to put strong direct pressure on her fundus and hold it for 15 minutes whenever she feels this pain.
   B. Inform Dee that abdominal pain is expected at this stage of her pregnancy and she should learn to adjust to it.
   C. Inquire about the specific nature and location of the pain Dee reported, since it could indicate a complication.
   D. Tell Dee to lie on her side at night to relieve the pressure on her intestinal tract and stomach.

6. Which of the following symptoms would the nurse expect to assess less commonly in early pregnancy?
   A. Braxton Hicks contractions
   B. Frequency of urination
   C. Ankle edema
   D. Varicosities

7. Tina is a heavy smoker (two packs per day) and is pregnant. Which of the following measures undertaken by Tina would indicate that a teaching plan for her had been most effective?
   A. She limited her cigarette smoking to one pack per day during her last months of pregnancy.
   B. She decreased her smoking by two cigarettes per day until she had stopped completely.
   C. She stated she will smoke only filtered cigarettes while she is pregnant.
   D. She voiced understanding that she will use nicotine gum and stop smoking immediately.

ALTERNATE FORMAT QUESTIONS

Fill in the Blank

Supply the missing term or the information requested.

1. Assessment of the pregnant woman concentrates on screening for the presence of ——— in the pregnant woman's environment and any abnormalities that might be occurring with the pregnancy.

2. Three environmental teratogens are metal and chemical hazards, ———, ——— and ———.

Multiple-Answer Multiple Choice

Circle the letter(s) corresponding to the appropriate answer(s). Select all that apply.

1. What are the common discomforts experienced during the first trimester of pregnancy?
   A. Hemorrhoids
   B. Breast tenderness
   C. Diarrhea
   D. Menstrual "spotting"
   E. Frequent urination

2. Select the symptoms that are viewed as signs of beginning labor.
   A. Depression
   B. Rupture of membrane
   C. Contractions
   D. Slight elevation in temperature
   E. Lightening

CHAPTER 12

Promoting Nutritional Health During Pregnancy

CHAPTER OVERVIEW

Chapter 12 provides an overview of the nutritional needs of a woman throughout pregnancy. The nutritional guidelines for pregnancy are reviewed. The use of the nursing process to plan and provide appropriate teaching related to nutritional health during pregnancy is explored.

LEARNING OBJECTIVES

After mastering the content in this chapter, you should be able to do the following:

1. Describe the requirements for healthy nutrition during pregnancy.
2. Assess a woman's nutrition during pregnancy.
3. Formulate nursing diagnoses related to nutritional concerns during pregnancy.
4. Develop expected outcomes to assist the pregnant woman to achieve optimal nutrition during pregnancy.
5. Plan health teaching strategies, such as ways to increase iron and calcium intake, to promote optimal nutritional intake during pregnancy.
6. Implement nursing care that encourages healthy nutritional practices during pregnancy.
7. Evaluate expected outcomes for achievement and effectiveness of nutritional care.
8. Identify National Health Goals related to nutrition and pregnancy that nurses can be instrumental in helping the nation achieve.
9. Identify areas related to nutrition and pregnancy that could benefit from additional nursing research or application of evidence-based practice.
10. Use critical thinking to analyze the effects of different life situations on nutrition patterns and ways nutritional health can be improved and family-centered.
11. Integrate nutrition knowledge with the nursing process to achieve quality maternal and child health nursing care.

KEY TERMS

body mass index
complete protein
Hawthorne effect
hypercholesterolemia
hyperplasia
hypertrophy
incomplete protein
lactase
obese
overweight
pica
pyrosis
underweight

■ Mastering the Information

MATCHING

Match the terms in Column I with a definition, example, or related statement from Column II. Place the letter corresponding to the answer in the space provided.

COLUMN I

1. ____Complete protein
2. ____Hyperplasia
3. ____Incomplete protein
4. ____Lactase
5. ____Linoleic acid
6. ____Obese
7. ____Phenylketonuria
8. ____Pica
9. ____Complementary proteins
10. ____Pyrosis

COLUMN II

a. A fatty oil that cannot be manufactured in the body from other sources
b. Foods containing fewer than eight of the essential amino acids
c. An abnormal craving for nonfood substances
d. A food containing all eight essential amino acids
e. An increase in the number of cells formed
f. Foods that when cooked together provide all eight amino acids
g. A burning sensation along the esophagus caused by decreased gastric motility
h. A woman weighing over 200 pounds, having a body mass index over 29, or being 50% above ideal body weight
i. The enzyme needed to break down milk sugar into glucose and galactose
j. An inability to convert an essential amino acid into tyrosine

SHORT ANSWER

Supply the missing term or the information requested.

1. Discuss the relationship between maternal dietary intake and fetal growth and development.
2. What factors may cause a woman to have decreased nutritional stores during pregnancy?
3. Discuss two types of food that should be avoided in pregnancy. Why should these foods be avoided?
4. Indicate the sources of the following substances and their significance for the pregnant woman: protein, calcium, fat, folic acid, iodine, iron.

■ Applying Your Knowledge

CASE STUDY

Ellen, age 16, is in her second trimester of pregnancy. She is at the clinic for her initial prenatal visit.

1. What are the most important initial assessments you would make before discussing nutritional needs with Ellen?
2. What nutritional intake behaviors do most adolescents exhibit that might make it difficult to promote adequate nutrition for Ellen and her fetus?
3. Compare the dietary instructions you might provide for a pregnant adolescent like Ellen with those for a pregnant woman over age 35.

CRITICAL INQUIRY EXERCISE

1. Prepare a 24-hour recall history using your own nutritional intake. Assess your dietary intake for adequacy. What changes would be necessary if you were pregnant?
2. What are five common foods served at fast-food restaurants that could be eaten to meet nutritional requirements? What are five foods that would be poor nutritional choices for the pregnant woman?

CRITICAL EXPLORATION

Perform a diet history on a pregnant adolescent woman and develop a teaching plan that addresses the nutritional needs of pregnancy.

■ Practicing for NCLEX

MULTIPLE-CHOICE QUESTIONS

Circle the letter that corresponds to the best answer for each question.

1. Which of the following measures undertaken by Dee would indicate that a teaching plan on nutrition during pregnancy had been effective?
   A. Plans a diet limiting protein intake to minimize metabolic waste during her last months of pregnancy
   B. Remains slim during the first 5 months of her pregnancy and small during the final months of pregnancy
   C. States she understands that, although she is obese, she should not diet to lose weight but should avoid eating empty calories
   D. Voices understanding that she should take over-the-counter vitamin and mineral preparations twice daily to supplement her diet

2. Pam is a 23-year-old single mother who has a 15-month-old and a 3-month-old who was premature; she had a miscarriage before the birth of her 3-month-old. Her diet history revealed that she likes to eat fish and chicken. Pam should be considered at nutritional risk because of her:
   A. Prior pregnancies
   B. Risky age group
   C. Single marital status
   D. Unusual food preferences

3. A woman with phenylketonuria should do which of the following?
   A. Avoid pregnancy, since it would aggravate her condition.
   B. Avoid food restrictions of any kind during her pregnancy.
   C. Return to a low-phenylalanine diet before becoming pregnant.
   D. Increase her intake of phenylalanine if she will breast-feed.

4. Which of the following would be an appropriate nursing intervention to help a woman with nausea and vomiting maintain adequate nutritional intake?
   A. Advise her to take daily laxatives to stimulate peristalsis and food digestion.
   B. Encourage her to eat meals before going to bed, when nausea is less severe.
   C. Suggest she eat foods that are high in fat to increase caloric intake.
   D. Teach her to refrain from eating for at least 6 hours prior to bedtime.

ALTERNATE FORMAT QUESTIONS

Fill in the Blank

Supply the missing term or the information requested.

1. A weight gain of ——— is currently recommended as an average weight gain in pregnancy.

2. Pregnant women who are vegetarians may lack vitamin ———, vitamin ———, and ——— in their diet.

3. Underweight women may need to increase their caloric intake by ——— to ——— calories above the calories ordinarily specified during pregnancy.

Multiple-Answer Multiple Choice

Circle the letter(s) corresponding to the appropriate answer(s). Select all that apply.

1. Which of the following foods would be most appropriate for the nurse to suggest a pregnant client consume if that client has low hemoglobin levels?
   A. Eggs
   B. Vegetable oils
   C. Milk
   D. Green leafy vegetables
   E. Organ meats

2. Bonnie, 3 months pregnant, has reported for her first prenatal visit. The nurse should instruct her to do which of the following?
   A. Eat foods rich in protein, iron, and other nutrients to provide an additional 300 calories each day.
   B. Increase her intake of carbohydrates (breads and sweets) to prevent protein metabolism.
   C. Eat small and frequent meals to increase absorption and decrease nausea.
   D. Eat whenever she feels hungry, because her body will let her know when she needs nutrients and extra calories.
   E. Limit intake of amino acids to prevent development of diabetic ketoacidosis.

CHAPTER 13

Preparation for Childbirth and Parenting

CHAPTER OVERVIEW

Chapter 13 addresses the woman who is preparing for the birth of a child. Physical and psychological readiness is addressed in terms of exercises and psychological techniques for pain control. The nursing interventions during the laboring process in the various types of birth settings are presented. The chapter presents a case study that describes principles pertinent to providing guidance to parents who may choose to participate in an alternative birth method.

LEARNING OBJECTIVES

After mastering the content in this chapter, you should be able to do the following:

1. Describe common alternative settings for birth and preparation necessary for childbirth and parenting.
2. Assess a couple for readiness for childbirth with regard to choice of birth attendant, preparation for labor, and setting.
3. Formulate nursing diagnoses related to preparation for childbirth and parenting.
4. Identify expected outcomes for the couple preparing for childbirth and parenting.
5. Plan nursing care, such as teaching exercises that are effective for strengthening abdominal and perineal muscles for childbirth.
6. Implement nursing care, such as supporting a woman during labor by the Lamaze method of prepared childbirth or helping a couple select and prepare for an alternative birth setting such as the home.
7. Evaluate outcome criteria for achievement and effectiveness of care.
8. Identify National Health Goals related to preparation for parenthood that nurses could be instrumental in helping the nation to achieve.
9. Identify areas related to preparation for childbirth that could benefit from additional nursing research or application of evidence-based practice.
10. Use critical thinking to analyze ways that birth can be made more family-centered through the use of prepared childbirth classes and alternative birth settings.
11. Integrate the principles of prepared childbirth with the nursing process to achieve quality maternal and child health nursing care.

KEY TERMS

alternative birthing center
birthing bed
birthing chair
birthing room
cleansing breath
conditioned reflexes
consciously controlled breathing
conscious relaxation
effleurage
gate control theory of pain perception
labor-delivery-recovery-postpartum room
labor-delivery-recovery room
Leboyer method
psychoprophylaxis
vaginal birth after cesarean birth

■ Mastering the Information

MATCHING

Match the terms in Column I with a definition, example, or related statement from Column II. Place the letter corresponding to the answer in the space provided.

COLUMN I

1. _____Imaging
2. _____Dick-Read method
3. _____Conditioned reflex
4. _____Tailor sitting
5. _____Squatting
6. _____Bradley method

COLUMN II

a. Measure that increases blood supply to the lower limbs and stretches the perineum
b. A physical response prompted by hearing a word or phrase
c. Method of childbirth based on the belief that birth is a natural process that should include the husband during the entire birthing process
d. Intense focusing on an object ("sensate focus"), inhibiting sensory input from reaching the cortex of the brain
e. Positioning the feet flat on the floor while stretching the perineal muscles
f. Method of childbirth based on the premise that fear leads to tension, which leads to pain

SHORT ANSWER

Supply the missing term or the information requested.

1. Describe the physiology of the following techniques of the gate control theory:
   A. Distraction
   B. Reduction of anxiety

2. Identify the advantages and disadvantages for the following birth settings: hospital, alternative birth center, home birth.

■ Applying Your Knowledge

CASE STUDY

Mrs. Virion, age 22, is interested in delivering her baby at home.

1. What factors would cause a woman to be considered a good candidate for a home birth?

2. What is considered to be the main advantage of a home birth?

3. State the expected outcomes when teaching Mrs. Virion how to perform the following exercises: abdominal contraction, pelvic floor contractions, and pelvic rocking.

CRITICAL INQUIRY EXERCISE

1. Develop a teaching plan for the techniques of perineal exercises. Include a proposed time schedule for implementing the exercises for a woman who works from 8 a.m. to 5 p.m.

2. Outline the main features of the popular Lamaze method of birthing. What behavioral characteristics would you look for in the family who would be most appropriate for this method?

CRITICAL EXPLORATION

1. Attend a prenatal class at a well-baby health clinic. Present an overview of childbirth methods and education principles; discuss the ultimate goal of childbirth. Then provide the names of some referral sources to the mothers so they may obtain more information on childbirth and parenting education.

2. Interview a couple who has recently become aware of their pregnancy. Discuss several alternative settings for the birth and emphasize the advantages and disadvantages of each.

■ Practicing for NCLEX

MULTIPLE-CHOICE QUESTIONS

Circle the letter that corresponds to the best answer for each question.

1. Effleurage, a technique used to displace pain, is described as:
   A. Light abdominal massage
   B. Focusing on an object to block sensory input
   C. The prophylaxis method
   D. The psychosexual method

2. In consciously controlled breathing methods, level 5 behaviors are defined as:
   A. Slow chest breathing at a rate of 6 to 12 breaths/minute
   B. Chest panting shallowly and continuously at a rate of 60 breaths/minute or more (during strong contractions)
   C. Pant-blow rhythm intermittently with forceful exhalations
   D. Light breathing and expanding the rib cage, at a rate of up to 40 breaths per minute (during transition contractions)

3. Flexing the lumbar spine can relieve backaches during pregnancy and early labor. This exercise is called:
   A. Kegel exercising
   B. Pelvic rocking
   C. Squatting
   D. Pelvic tailoring

ALTERNATE FORMAT QUESTIONS

Fill in the Blank

Supply the missing term or the information requested.

1. Encouraging progressive breathing, including conscious relaxation, is called ————.
2. ——— is light abdominal massage in conjunction with breathing exercises.
3. ——— are used with repetition to strengthen the floor of the perineum.
4. Prevention of pain during birth by use of the mind is called ————.

Multiple-Answer Multiple Choice

Circle the letter(s) corresponding to the appropriate answer(s). Select all that apply.

1. Which of the following would be most appropriate to do for the birth environment in preparation for the Leboyer method?
   A. Spraying the birthing room just before delivery with insecticides to reduce the microorganism counts
   B. Raising the temperature of the room slightly just before the birth
   C. Keeping the birthing room as cool as the hospital delivery room to reduce the chance of bacteria growth
   D. Darkening the room after the birth and assessment to lessen the impact of the environmental change on the newborn
   E. Adjusting the room to operate as a negative-pressure room to protect against environmental infections

4. Which of the following instructions would be most appropriate to help a pregnant woman avoid orthostatic hypertension?
   A. Upon awakening, sitting upright for several minutes before standing
   B. Holding her breath while exercising
   C. Hyperextending her lower back
   D. Getting up slowly from the floor after exercising
   E. Rolling from side to side during exercise

CHAPTER 14

High-Risk Pregnancy: The Woman with a Preexisting or Newly Acquired Illness

CHAPTER OVERVIEW

Chapter 14 provides an overview of various systemic conditions that can result in a client assuming a high-risk pregnancy status. The effects of various physical illnesses on the woman and her fetus during pregnancy stages are discussed. The use of the nursing process to plan and provide care for the client, the fetus, and the family involved in a high-risk pregnancy is explored.

LEARNING OBJECTIVES

After mastering the content in this chapter, you should be able to do the following:

1. Define high-risk pregnancy, including factors that contribute to its development.
2. Describe common illnesses such as cardiovascular disease, diabetes mellitus, or renal and blood disorders that can result in complications when they exist with pregnancy.
3. Assess the woman with an illness during pregnancy for changes occurring because of the pregnancy.
4. List nursing diagnoses related to the effect of a preexisting or newly acquired illness on pregnancy.
5. Identify appropriate outcomes that will contribute to a safe pregnancy outcome when illness occurs with pregnancy (e.g., planning ways a woman can get more rest).
6. Plan nursing care for the woman with an illness during pregnancy (e.g., teaching insulin administration to a woman newly diagnosed with gestational diabetes).
7. Implement nursing care for the woman when illness complicates pregnancy.
8. Evaluate expected outcomes to determine achievement and effectiveness of care.
9. Identify National Health Goals related to complications of pregnancy that nurses can be instrumental in helping the nation achieve.
10. Identify areas related to illness and pregnancy that could benefit from additional nursing research or application of evidence-based practice.
11. Use critical thinking to analyze ways that nursing care can remain family-centered when a preexisting illness is present or a newly acquired illness develops.
12. Integrate knowledge of high-risk pregnancy and the nursing process to achieve quality maternal and child health nursing care.

KEY TERMS

deep vein thrombosis
glucose tolerance test
glycosuria
glycosylated hemoglobin
high-risk pregnancy
hyperglycemia
hypoglycemia
insulin pump
megaloblastic anemia
orthopnea
paroxysmal nocturnal dyspnea
peripartal cardiomyopathy
proteinuria
sexually transmitted disease

■ Mastering the Information

MATCHING

Match the terms in Column I with a definition, example, or related statement from Column II. Place the letter corresponding to the answer in the space provided.

COLUMN I

1. ____Functional heart murmur
2. ____Paroxysmal nocturnal dyspnea
3. ____Megaloblastic anemia

4. ____Left heart failure
5. ____Pyelonephritis
6. ____Hiatal hernia
7. ____Scoliosis
8. ____Systemic lupus erythematosus
9. ____Pseudoanemia
10. ____*Chlamydia trachomatis*

COLUMN II

a. Occurs when mitral valve stenosis or insufficiency or aortic coarctation causes a decrease in cardiac output and back pressure to the lungs
b. A normal decrease in the red blood cell count due to the expanded blood volume of pregnancy
c. An innocent, transient escape of fluid through heart valves due to increased blood flow past valves that can occur during pregnancy
d. Low blood levels with enlarged red blood cells related to folic acid deficiency
e. A multisystem connective tissue disease that may result in acute nephritis
f. A portion of the stomach extended through the diaphragm that can result in inability to eat due to heartburn
g. Lateral curvature of the spine that may cause pelvic distortion that can interfere with childbirth
h. Suddenly waking during the night with severe shortness of breath
i. Kidney infection that can result in premature labor or rupture of membranes
j. The most common vaginal infection seen during pregnancy

COLUMN I

1. _____Viral hepatitis
2. _____Human immunodeficiency virus
3. _____Schizophrenia
4. _____Tonic-clonic seizures
5. _____Burns
6. _____Celiotomy

COLUMN II

A. Exploratory abdominal surgery performed to detect bleeding due to traumatic injury
B. Danger to mother and fetus due to carbon monoxide and fluid/electrolyte losses
C. Jaundice occurs as a late symptom.
D. Maternal infection with this virus requires active interactions to reduce fetal exposure to maternal blood.
E. Treatment with teratogenic medication may be necessary.
F. Possible anoxia occurring from spasm of chest muscles

SHORT ANSWER

Supply the missing term or the information requested.

1. List one example each of psychological, social, and physical factors that can cause a pregnancy to be categorized as high risk during the pre-pregnancy, pregnancy, and labor and delivery periods.

2. Describe how pregnancy can cause a woman to develop a urinary tract infection.

3. Discuss the key issues that should be included in a teaching plan for a pregnant woman who is a diabetic or who develops diabetes during pregnancy. Address diet, exercise, insulin, and glucose monitoring.

4. Describe one safety precaution in each of three areas—home, work, and automobile safety—that may be taken by a pregnant woman to prevent accidental injury.

5. Describe the procedure for airway clearance on a pregnant choking victim.

■ Applying Your Knowledge

CASE STUDY

Melinda Jaffe is a 28-year-old mother of two, ages 5 and 3. Melinda is in for her second prenatal visit. She is 5 months pregnant and has a history of congestive heart failure secondary to valve disease from childhood rheumatic fever.

1. What is the most dangerous time in the pregnancy for a woman with heart disease? Why?

2. How might the fact that Melinda has two young children affect her risk for complications from her heart disease? What nursing interventions would you plan?

3. How might Melinda's risk of complications be different if she had had valve replacement surgery years prior to the pregnancy?

CRITICAL INQUIRY EXERCISE

1. What would be the major points you would include in a teaching plan for adolescents that addresses the effects of sexually transmitted diseases on a fetus or on an infant after childbirth?

2. In what way, if any, would your teaching plan differ for an insulin-dependent diabetic who became pregnant, and for a pregnant woman who developed gestational diabetes?

CRITICAL EXPLORATION

While on a postpartal clinical unit, review the chart of a client with diabetes. Note the prenatal history, course of the pregnancy for glucose regulation, any complications experienced, postpartal glucose control, and status of the newborn.

■ Practicing for NCLEX

MULTIPLE-CHOICE QUESTIONS

Circle the letter that corresponds to the best answer for each question.

1. Melle, 12 years old, is 2 months pregnant and has a history of heart disease. Which of the following is true about her risk factors for high-risk pregnancy?
   A. Good nutrition and exercise will eliminate any added risk factors Melle may have for complications.
   B. Melle's heart condition will not affect her pregnancy, since she has not reached adolescence.
   C. Melle's youth will protect her from many problems experienced by older women with heart disease.
   D. Both Melle's age and heart condition will place her at risk for complications during pregnancy.

2. Which of the following could be included in the outcome criteria for a client with the nursing diagnosis "Ineffective tissue perfusion (fetal or maternal) related to maternal cardiovascular disease"?
   A. Bed rest is maintained at home after the 36th week of gestation.
   B. Fetal heart rate will remain between 120 and 160 beats a minute.
   C. Jugular vein distention is evident when lying at 45 degrees.
   D. Maternal blood pressure is maintained above 150 systolic.

3. When planning care for a pregnant woman with heart disease, the nurse should do which of the following?
   A. Assess all complaints of fatigue and note any accompanying dyspnea or pulmonary congestion.
   B. Discourage the mother from taking any medications during pregnancy, since they will affect the baby.
   C. Instruct the client to eat as much food as desired to promote maximum fetal and maternal nutrition.
   D. Plan an exercise schedule to prevent thrombus formation during labor.

4. Which of the following interventions should be implemented with caution when caring for a postpartal woman who has heart disease or hypertensive vascular disease?
   A. Administering prenatal vitamins
   B. Ensuring early ambulation with antiembolism stockings
   C. Encouraging bulk and high fiber content in the diet
   D. Suggesting oral contraceptives as a birth control method

5. Pregnant women with venous thromboembolic disease:
   A. Are at risk for death from a pulmonary embolism.
   B. Must have oral fluids restricted throughout the pregnancy.
   C. Should receive heparin as soon as their labor begins.
   D. Need teaching to keep their legs crossed at the knee when sitting.

6. Clients with megaloblastic anemia should be encouraged to do which of the following?
   A. Avoid pregnancy, since they cannot carry the baby to term.
   B. Avoid excessive fluid intake, which has caused this hemodilution.
   C. Take over-the-counter multivitamins.
   D. Take the prescribed folic acid supplements.

7. When planning care for a pregnant client with sickle-cell anemia, the nurse might establish which of the following outcome criteria? The client:
   A. Lies on her back in a semi-Fowler's position when sleeping
   B. Rests with her legs elevated when sitting in a chair
   C. Reports intent to get a sickle-cell antigen shot after delivery
   D. States understanding of need to limit fluid intake to 16 ounces/day

8. Clients with chronic renal disease or who have had kidney transplants may have difficulty in pregnancy for which of the following reasons?
   A. Fetal waste products must be excreted in addition to maternal waste products.
   B. Hormones released in pregnancy can cause rejection of the transplant.
   C. Increased glomerular filtration rate causes decreased serum creatinine level.
   D. Steroids may cause excessive fetal growth stimulation.

9. Measures the nurse should implement for the pregnant client with rheumatoid arthritis include which of the following?
   A. Discussing the woman's intent to breast-feed so that medications can be changed if necessary
   B. Instructing the woman to increase her intake of aspirin 2 weeks prior to term to offset the decrease in corticosteroids
   C. Encouraging the woman to contact her physician for a higher dosage, if methotrexate is prescribed
   D. Assessing the client each week to monitor for blood clots due to salicylate ingestion

10. Teresa, who is at 20 weeks' gestation, has been diagnosed with acute appendicitis. She expresses concern that the doctor is going to perform surgery. The nurse could explain which of the following?
    A. Delivery of the baby with a cesarean birth at this point would be safer than trying to complete the pregnancy.
    B. Since the appendix cannot be removed at this stage of the pregnancy without disruption of the pregnancy, an abortion is necessary.
    C. If she prefers, the doctor can delay removal of the appendix until later in the pregnancy.
    D. Peritonitis could result from rupture of the appendix and would be dangerous for both mother and child.

11. Which of the following evaluation data would indicate that the nurse's teaching plan for the pregnant client with cholecystitis had been effective?
    A. Aching occurs only in the right epigastrium after eating.
    B. Jaundice and pain remain absent throughout the pregnancy.
    C. The client prepares a menu that is fat-free.
    D. The client reports ingestion of high-cholesterol foods.

12. A pregnant woman diagnosed with diabetes should be instructed to do which of the following to control her glucose level?
    A. Discontinue insulin injections until pregnancy is completed, since hormones will regulate glucose levels.
    B. Ingest a smaller amount of food prior to sleep to prevent nocturnal hyperglycemia.
    C. Notify the physician if she is unable to eat due to nausea and vomiting.
    D. Prepare foods with increased fat content to provide needed calories.

13. After delivery, a diabetic woman might need to do which of the following?
    A. Change to oral hypoglycemia agents, which will control glucose levels more effectively than insulin.
    B. Bottle-feed her infant, since insulin received through breast-feeding may cause hypoglycemia in the child.
    C. Receive no insulin during the immediate postpartal period, since insulin resistance is gone.
    D. Take medications to decrease uterine hypertonicity if hydramnios was present during pregnancy.

14. Which of the following data would support a diagnosis of "Compromised family coping related to poor communication between partners or potentially abusive father"?
    A. The woman and her husband always report together for prenatal visits.
    B. The woman states concern that her baby may not have a good heartbeat because she "fell down recently."
    C. You notice that the woman wears a low-cut dress or blouse at each prenatal visit.
    D. Examination reveals that fetal heart tones and fundal height indicate the baby might weigh over 8 pounds.

15. When preparing for a postmortem delivery, the nurse should do which of the following?
    A. Begin the oxytocin drip and regulate it slowly to aid vaginal delivery.
    B. Determine if the pregnancy is earlier than 24 weeks' gestation, since a young fetus will be more likely to survive.
    C. Obtain equipment necessary for immediate resuscitation of the newborn.
    D. Prepare a consent form, since the surgery cannot be performed without a consent.

16. Which of the following nursing interventions would be appropriate when caring for a pregnant client who has the nursing diagnosis "Ineffective tissue perfusion related to blood loss through a gunshot or stab wound"?
    A. Encourage a sitting position that will maintain pressure to abdominal organs and control bleeding.
    B. Prepare to administer antihypotensive drugs, which will cause peripheral vasoconstriction and maintain blood pressure.
    C. Recognize that since pregnant women have higher-than-normal fluid volume, small losses of blood will have severe vascular effects.
    D. Position the client in a side-lying position to decrease vena caval pressure.

17. Nursing measures implemented with a pregnant client who has experienced trauma would include which of the following?
    A. Concentrating on controlling the client's anxiety first and foremost
    B. Monitoring for other signs of shock, since the client's skin might not be cold and clammy
    C. Positioning the client on her back in reverse Trendelenburg's
    D. Recognizing that a heart rate increase of 15 to 20 beats above the nonpregnant rate indicates hypovolemia

18. Pregnant women should be taught to be careful to avoid accidental injury. They are prone to falls for which of the following reasons?
    A. Additional weight from pregnancy may disturb balance when walking.
    B. Fetal activity stimulates the nerves of the legs and causes weakness.
    C. High levels of hormones often impair judgment, resulting in reckless behavior.
    D. Increased adrenaline released during pregnancy causes women to move faster than usual.

ALTERNATE FORMAT QUESTIONS

Fill in the Blank

Supply the missing term or the information requested.

1. ——— ——— ——— could cause cardiac failure, anemia, and hypertensive vascular disease to result in fetal distress or low birthweight.
2. Three factors in pregnancy that can result in venous thromboembolic disease are ——— ——— and ———.

Multiple-Answer Multiple Choice

Circle the letter(s) corresponding to the appropriate answer(s). Select all that apply.

1. Identify the common sexually transmitted diseases that may affect the newborn.
   A. Herpes simplex 1
   B. Trichomoniasis
   C. Cellulitis
   D. Gonorrhea
   E. Chlamydia
2. Which of the following is an appropriate outcome criterion for the pregnant client who has seizures as a result of childhood meningitis? The client:
   A. Demonstrates ability to recognize the Moro reflex as an early indication of fetal seizures
   B. Requires no supplemental oxygen administration during convulsions
   C. States understanding that her child is not certain to have seizures just because she developed the condition
   D. Refrains from taking anticonvulsant medications during the first trimester to prevent congenital defects
   E. Understands that chromosomal defects are not the etiology of her seizures

CHAPTER 15

High-Risk Pregnancy: The Woman Who Develops a Complication of Pregnancy

CHAPTER OVERVIEW

Chapter 15 discusses the complications that can occur during pregnancy and the effects these complications have on the woman and her family. The use of the nursing process to plan and provide care for the client and family under these circumstances is explored.

LEARNING OBJECTIVES

After mastering the content in this chapter, you should be able to do the following:

1. Describe complications of pregnancy that place the pregnant woman and her fetus at high risk.
2. Assess the woman who is experiencing a complication of pregnancy.
3. Formulate nursing diagnoses that address the needs of the woman and her family experiencing a complication of pregnancy.
4. Identify outcomes to minimize the risks to the pregnant woman and her fetus.
5. Plan nursing interventions to meet the needs and promote optimal outcome for the woman and her family.
6. Implement nursing actions specific to the woman who has developed a complication of pregnancy.
7. Evaluate outcomes for effectiveness and achievement.
8. Identify National Health Goals related to complications of pregnancy and specific measures nurses can take to help the nation achieve these goals.
9. Identify areas of nursing care related to high-risk pregnancy that could benefit from additional nursing research or the application of evidence-based practice.
10. Use critical thinking to analyze ways that nurses can help prevent complications of pregnancy.
11. Integrate knowledge of complications of pregnancy with the nursing process to achieve quality maternal and child health nursing care.

KEY TERMS

abortion
ankle clonus
cervical cerclage
cervical ripening
chorioamnionitis
complete miscarriage
couvelaire uterus
early pregnancy failure
eclampsia
ectopic pregnancy
erythroblastosis fetalis
gestational trophoblastic disease
HELLP syndrome
hemolytic disease of the newborn
hydramnios
incomplete miscarriage
isoimmunization miscarriage
placenta previa
post-term pregnancy
preeclampsia
premature cervical dilatation
premature separation of the placenta
preterm labor
preterm rupture of the membranes
pseudocyesis
recurrent pregnancy loss
Rh incompatibility
tocolytic agent

■ Mastering the Information

MATCHING

Match the terms in Column I with a definition, example, or related statement from Column II. Place the letter corresponding to the answer in the space provided.

COLUMN I

1. _____Placenta previa
2. _____Isoimmunization
3. _____Cervical cerclage
4. _____Imminent miscarriage
5. _____Erythroblastosis

6. ____Abruptio placentae
7. ____Pseudocyesis
8. ____Late spontaneous miscarriage
9. ____Eclampsia
10. ____Gestational trophoblastic disease (hydatidiform mole)
11. ____Ectopic pregnancy

COLUMN II

a. An interruption of pregnancy (natural causes) occuring between the 16th and 24th week
b. Implantation occurring outside the uterine cavity
c. Proliferation and degeneration of the trophoblast villi
d. Low implantation of the placenta
e. Pregnancy-induced hypertension, proteinuria, and cerebral edema with seizure
f. Purse-string sutures applied to prevent recurrence of premature dilation and fetal expulsion (loss)
g. Event occurring when an Rh-negative woman is exposed to Rh-positive fetal blood
h. Premature separation of the placenta
i. Vaginal bleeding with uterine contractions and cervical dilation prior to fetal viability
j. Hemolytic disease of the newborn
k. Amenorrhea, nausea, and enlargement of the abdomen occuring in a nonpregnant woman

IDENTIFICATION

For each of the pregnancy complications listed below, indicate when it usually occurs with the letter "A" for first trimester, "B" for second trimester, and "C" for third trimester.

1. ——— Placenta previa
2. ——— Spontaneous miscarriage
3. ——— Hydatidiform mole
4. ——— Abruptio placentae
5. ——— Incompetent cervix
6. ——— Ectopic pregnancy

SHORT ANSWER

Supply the missing term or the information requested.

1. An unplanned interruption of pregnancy before the fetus is viable is the definition of what condition?

2. Pregnancy in which implantation occurs outside the uterine cavity is the definition of what condition?

3. Hypertension of pregnancy that involves hemolysis, high liver enzymes, and low platelet levels is the definition of what condition?

4. Hypertension of pregnancy with BP that is elevated 30 mm Hg systolic or 15 mm Hg diastolic above prepregnancy values is the definition of what condition?

5. Excessive amniotic fluid formation is the definition of what condition?

6. Briefly explain why it is important to determine the week of pregnancy at which bleeding began to occur.

7. Contrast the symptoms noted by a woman with a normal pregnancy with those that may be noted by a woman with an ectopic pregnancy.

8. Discuss the use of heparin to treat disseminated intravascular coagulation.

9. Explain how a teaching plan for a client with multiple gestation would differ from a plan for a client with single gestation in the following areas: activity, nutrition, complications, and role changes.

■ Applying Your Knowledge

CASE STUDY

Danielle is a 38-year-old secretary who is pregnant with her first child. She is 5-foot-6 and weighs 210 pounds. When she presents at the clinic for her seventh-month visit, the nurse notes her blood pressure is 148/92. She states she has had ankle edema for several months now but lately has noticed swelling in her face and hands.

1. What evaluation data would indicate that the nursing interventions to help control mild preeclampsia had been effective?

2. What symptoms might signal the development of pregnancy-induced hypertension? How would you teach a client to monitor for them?

3. What nursing measures would you implement for a client with pregnancy-induced hypertension (eclampsia)? What activities would you avoid?

CRITICAL EXPLORATION

Monitor the care of a client with preeclampsia or eclampsia. Note the nursing care provided and medications used.

■ Practicing for NCLEX

MULTIPLE-CHOICE QUESTIONS

Circle the letter that corresponds to the best answer for each question.

1. Mrs. Dean is 2 months pregnant and has a history of two spontaneous miscarriages. Which of the following assessments indicates a potential for a third miscarriage?
   A. Lab results revealing an elevation in protein-bound iodine
   B. Dietary intake indicating 300 more calories than eaten by the nonpregnant female
   C. Reports of exposure to a child with rubella over a period of time
   D. Nervous, anxious behavior noted during the prenatal visits

2. The nurse monitoring a client who is experiencing a miscarriage episode must consider which of the following facts?
   A. Miscarriages occurring before the sixth week of pregnancy often result in severe bleeding and hypovolemia.
   B. A D&C can be performed to prevent a threatened miscarriage from advancing to an imminent miscarriage.
   C. A missed miscarriage will result in no expulsion of blood or fetal material until the fetus actually dies.
   D. Incomplete miscarriages present a greater potential for hemorrhage than do complete miscarriages.

3. If an Rh-negative woman experiences a miscarriage during her first pregnancy, she should be instructed to do which of the following?
   A. Adopt children, since future pregnancies will result in future miscarriages.
   B. Avoid pregnancy for the next year to permit a decrease in Rh antigens.
   C. Consume high doses of vitamin D and vitamin K to prevent anemia.
   D. Receive Rh(D antigen) immune globulin (RhIG) to prevent the buildup of antibodies.

4. When assessing a woman who is suspected of having an ectopic pregnancy, the nurse would report which of the following as a risk factor?
   A. A history of using intrauterine devices for birth control
   B. Nausea and vomiting during early pregnancy
   C. A soft, nontender abdomen with active bowel sounds
   D. Absence of vaginal bleeding or menstrual flow

5. Which of the following findings might be noted in a client with a hydatidiform mole?
   A. False-negative blood test results for pregnancy
   B. Fetal heart tones that are louder and faster than normal
   C. Marked (extreme) nausea and vomiting noted in early pregnancy
   D. Uterine growth occurring more slowly than in normal pregnancy

6. Which of the following nursing diagnoses may be indicated for a client diagnosed and treated for hydatidiform mole?
   A. Imbalanced nutrition, more than body requirements related to increased appetite
   B. Fluid volume excess related to polycythemia due to drug therapy
   C. Impaired adjustment related to incomplete grieving of lost pregnancy
   D. Ineffective family coping related to poor bonding with newborn

7. Dee Ball is admitted with placenta previa with 75% coverage of the cervical os. The fetus is at 35 weeks' gestation. Which of the following nursing measures should be implemented?
   A. Encourage Ms. Ball to lie on her back as much as possible.
   B. Instruct Ms. Ball to use a tampon to halt the vaginal bleeding.
   C. Obtain oxygen equipment to keep on standby in case of fetal distress.
   D. Teach Ms. Ball the importance of limiting stair-climbing.

8. Postmature pregnancy is dangerous to the fetus in which of the following ways?
   A. The fetus will suffer from decreased blood perfusion.
   B. Fetal inhalation results in aspiration of amniotic fluid.
   C. Hydramnios leading to decreased fetal circulation will occur.
   D. Microcephaly may result in increased biparietal diameter.

9. Which of the following is true about Rh incompatibility?
   A. If the mother is Rh negative and the father is homozygous Rh positive, the child will have a 50% chance of being Rh negative.
   B. If the mother is Rh negative and the father is heterozygous for the trait, 100% of the children can be expected to be Rh positive.
   C. The Rh-positive fetus inside of an Rh-negative mother is perceived as a foreign agent and stimulates the formation of antibodies.
   D. Women who are Rh negative and experience miscarriage of an Rh-positive fetus will not develop antibodies to foreign Rh antigen.

10. The client going through labor who knows her child will be stillborn will likely experience which of the following emotions?
    A. Relief that the pregnancy will be terminated early and she can begin to try again to have a baby
    B. Delight that she will not have to carry the heavy baby to term
    C. Grief at the loss of her infant and her inability to carry a pregnancy to term
    D. Confidence in her ability to conceive a child that will be viable

ALTERNATE FORMAT QUESTIONS

Fill in the Blank

Supply the missing term or the information requested.

1. The two main causes of bleeding during the second trimester are ———— and ————.
2. Sudden placental separation from the uterus with bleeding is called ————.

Multiple-Answer Multiple Choice

Circle the letter(s) corresponding to the appropriate answer(s). Select all that apply.

1. Which of the following would be cause for concern if it were noted during a prenatal assessment in the third trimester?
   A. Frequent painless urination
   B. Fetal movement after eating
   C. Meconium appearing as vaginal discharge
   D. Back pain and problems finding a comfortable sleeping position
   E. An additional, severe pain occurring with each contraction

2. Which of the following observations might indicate fetal death?
   A. Failure of labor to begin before the 42nd week of gestation
   B. Reports that the fetus has been very lazy and has not moved or kicked
   C. Sonogram readings that reveal a rapid heart rate and rhythm
   D. Absence of fetal movement in the period of pregnancy after quickening
   E. Dark green sticky substance noted when membranes ruptured

CHAPTER 16

Home Care of the Pregnant Client

CHAPTER OVERVIEW

Chapter 16 discusses the usual health concerns that require home care nursing during pregnancy and the appropriate nursing actions required to identify and assist a client in the home setting. Medication therapy is reviewed and nursing implications related to the administration of medications and patient/family teaching are outlined. The use of the nursing process to plan and provide appropriate care and teaching to assist the woman to care for herself and avoid complications is discussed.

LEARNING OBJECTIVES

After mastering the content in this chapter, you should be able to do the following:

1. Describe common health concerns requiring home care during pregnancy.
2. Assess the pregnant woman receiving home care.
3. Formulate nursing diagnoses related to care of the pregnant client at home.
4. Identify expected outcomes for the woman and family requiring home care.
5. Plan nursing care to meet the needs of the pregnant home care client.
6. Implement nursing care to meet the needs of the pregnant home care client.
7. Evaluate outcomes for effectiveness and achievement of a satisfying experience for a woman and her family.
8. Identify National Health Goals related to home care during pregnancy that nurses can help the nation achieve.
9. Identify areas of home care nursing that could benefit from additional nursing research or application of evidence-based practice.
10. Use critical thinking to analyze how home care influences family functioning, and develop ways to make nursing care more family-centered.
11. Integrate knowledge of home care with the nursing process to achieve quality maternal and child health nursing care.

KEY TERMS

home care
perinatal home care
skilled home nursing care

■ Mastering the Information

MATCHING

Match the terms in column I with a definition, example, or related statement from Column II. Place the letter corresponding to the answer in the space provided.

COLUMN I

1. _____Total parenteral nutrition
2. _____Perinatal home care
3. _____Post-visit planning
4. _____Skilled home nursing care

COLUMN II

a. Provision or supervision of care of a pregnant woman in the home by a home or community health care agency
b. A method of supplying complete nutrition and fluid to women with hyperemesis gravidarum that may be administered in the home setting
c. Nursing care provided in the home that includes physician-prescribed procedures such as dressing changes
d. Documentation, communication, and evaluation of client's future needs

SHORT ANSWER

Supply the missing term or the information requested.

1. When obtaining the health history and performing a physical exam in the client's home environment, the nurse must provide ——— and maintain ———.

2. If the home situation becomes unsafe while the nurse is visiting, the nurse should ———, and if the nurse and client are in danger the nurse should ——— the ——— ——— ——— for help.

3. A major portion of planning for home care involves reviewing with the woman and her family exactly what will be ——— of them and what ——— ——— ——— from you.

4. Discuss how nurses can be instrumental in helping the nation achieve National Health Goals related to prevention of preterm birth.

■ Applying Your Knowledge

CASE STUDY

Peg Waters, age 32, is admitted onto your unit. She is pregnant with her first child. Her husband is present and they both appear anxious because Peg has gone into labor in her 36th week of gestation.

1. Peg states, "I don't know how I'm going to manage staying at home and not working." What would the nurse's best response be, and why?

2. If Peg used intravenous medication to control premature labor, what would she need to know to manage her medication?

3. What key points would you explain to Peg to prepare her for delivery of a preterm infant if her labor is not halted?

CRITICAL INQUIRY EXERCISE

1. What key points would you address in a teaching plan for an adolescent who is on home care because she is experiencing preterm labor in her 32nd week of gestation? How would this plan differ for a 28-year-old woman? A 38-year-old woman?

2. You are supervising an unlicensed assistive personnel (UAP) in home care for a pregnant client. What are some areas you would discuss with the UAP before the first client visit?

CRITICAL EXPLORATION

Accompany a home health care nurse on one or more visits to a home-bound preterm labor patient. What are the major assessments and interventions made by the nurse? What changes would you make in the patient's regimen, if any, based on your observations?

■ Practicing for NCLEX

MULTIPLE-CHOICE QUESTIONS

Circle the letter that corresponds to the best answer for each question.

1. When planning a home visit, the nurse should do which of the following?
   A. Keep his or her schedule, destination, and travel route confidential to protect client privacy.
   B. Learn the location of public phones in the neighborhood.
   C. Drop in to visit the client on occasion to observe the family in a realistic state.
   D. Drive straight home if he or she suspects someone is following him or her.

2. Disadvantages of home care for a pregnant woman include which of the following?
   A. Care is done in the client's home.
   B. Family members are included in the plan of care.
   C. The pregnant patient assumes a greater responsibility for monitoring her condition.
   D. Family interactions, values, and priorities are more obvious than in a health care setting.

3. Which of the following is accurate instruction the nurse might need to provide to the pregnant woman receiving home care?
   A. To promote elimination, the woman should avoid high-fiber foods.
   B. When monitoring uterine contractions, the woman should count and time the contractions for 10 minutes.
   C. The woman should alternate arms with each reading when monitoring her blood pressure.
   D. Serial fundal height measurements should be taken at the same location each time.

4. Health teaching during a home care visit:
   A. Provides more opportunities for one-on-one teaching than in a health care agency
   B. Would not involve childbirth education, since formal classes are available
   C. Should not intrude into home activities such as food planning
   D. Involves instructing the woman to avoid all medications unless the nurse is present

5. Jackie's husband states he wants to help his wife, who is being treated at home for preterm labor. You could instruct him to do which of the following?
   A. Walk with Jackie two times each day to help her maintain adequate exercise to prevent thrombus formation.
   B. Restrict Jackie's intake of fluids to four glasses daily to prevent pulmonary edema.
   C. Remind Jackie to monitor fetal movements once a week to watch for fetal hyperactivity.
   D. Assume responsibility for childcare and household duties to help Jackie maintain strict bed rest.

ALTERNATE FORMAT QUESTIONS

Fill in the Blank

Supply the missing term or the information requested.

1. The nurse should plan visits at times that are convenient for the family in order not to disrupt __________________________________.

2. Women on home care should be evaluated every ___ days to see if their risk level has changed.

Multiple-Answer Multiple Choice

Circle the letter(s) corresponding to the appropriate answer(s). Select all that apply.

1. Priority assessments of the client at home would include:
   A. Health history
   B. Political views
   C. Mental status
   D. Activities and rest pattern
   E. Preference for birth control
   F. Accuracy of self-assessments
   G. Professional goals
   H. Transportation to follow-up appointments

2. Priority assessments of the home environment would include:
   A. Presence of telephone
   B. Safety of house for home care
   C. Color scheme for baby room
   D. Rodents or insects in the home
   E. Adequate water and heat
   F. Sufficient maternity clothing
   G. Refrigeration facilities
   H. Presence of father in the home

CHAPTER 17

High-Risk Pregnancy: A Woman with Special Needs

CHAPTER OVERVIEW

Chapter 17 discusses nursing care related to care of a woman with special needs during pregnancy. The needs of an adolescent, a woman over age 35, a woman with a physical handicap, and a woman with a drug dependency during pregnancy are reviewed. The use of the nursing process to plan and provide appropriate teaching for a woman with special needs throughout pregnancy is explored.

LEARNING OBJECTIVES

After mastering the content in this chapter, you should be able to do the following:

1. Identify the characteristics of a pregnant woman who has special needs.
2. Describe the risks of pregnancy for a woman with special needs.
3. Assess a woman with special needs during pregnancy.
4. State nursing diagnoses related to pregnancy for a woman with special needs.
5. Identify expected outcomes for a pregnant woman with special needs.
6. Plan nursing care to address the special growth and development needs of an adolescent and a woman over age 40 and the specific strengths and weaknesses of a woman who is physically or cognitively challenged or drug dependent during pregnancy.
7. Implement nursing care for a woman with special needs.
8. Evaluate outcomes to ensure that goals for care have been achieved.
9. Identify National Health Goals related to a woman with a special need that nurses can be instrumental in helping the nation to achieve.
10. Identify areas related to care of a woman with special needs during pregnancy that would benefit from additional nursing research or application of evidence-based practice.
11. Use critical thinking to analyze ways that nursing care of a pregnant woman with a special need can be optimally family-centered.
12. Integrate knowledge of risks of pregnancy with age extremes, drug use, and physical or cognitive challenges with the nursing process to achieve quality maternal and child health nursing care.

KEY TERMS

autonomic dysreflexia
emancipated minor
substance dependent

■ Mastering the Information

MATCHING

Match the terms in column I with a definition, example, or related statement from Column II. Place the letter corresponding to the answer in the space provided.

COLUMN I

1. ____Autonomic dysreflexia
2. ____Substance dependent
3. ____Cephalopelvic disproportion
4. ____Credé maneuver
5. ____Day history
6. ____Egocentric phenomenon
7. ____Nest-building behavior
8. ____Postpartal hemorrhage
9. ____Striae
10. ____Varicosities

COLUMN II

a. Complication associated with pregnant adolescents and women over 35 due to overdistention of the uterus or decreased uterine contractility
b. Pregnancy change that will probably fade from the adolescent's body following pregnancy
c. Written account of nutrition, sleep, daily activity, use of drugs, and support/friendships of the pregnant adolescent
d. A complication that may occur in a pregnant adolescent due to incomplete pelvic growth, necessitating a cesarean birth
e. Symptoms include severe hypertension, throbbing headache, nausea, bradycardia, skin flushing, and profuse diaphoresis in a woman with a high spinal cord injury.
f. The development of withdrawal symptoms following discontinuation of a substance
g. Common problem possibly prevented by resting daily with feet elevated and sleeping in Sims position to decrease venous congestion
h. Evidence of this may not be noted in women over 35 until after amniocentesis results determine the baby is healthy.
i. An adolescent's belief that although she is sexually active she won't become pregnant
j. Pressing the upper anterior surface of the bladder to constrict and empty it; can be used by pregnant women with no sensation of voiding

SHORT ANSWER

Supply the missing term or the information requested.

1. Name three factors that have contributed to the inability to stop teenage pregnancies.

2. Name three physical conditions that a pregnant adolescent is at high risk for developing.

3. Explain how nurses can be instrumental in helping the nation achieve the goal of reducing pregnancy among girls aged 17 and younger.

4. Discuss nursing responsibilities relative to child safety for the pregnant woman who is experiencing moderate or severe cognitive challenges.

5. Discuss the reasons a pregnant woman with drug dependency might not comply with a prenatal visitation schedule or proper diet.

■ Applying Your Knowledge

CASE STUDY

Bertha, age 16, has a T1 spinal injury due to an automobile accident 2 years ago. She is 4 months pregnant and is in for her second prenatal visit.

1. What are some of the major areas you would assess to determine priorities in planning care for Bertha?

2. In what ways will Bertha's age add to the complications normally present for a pregnant woman with a spinal cord injury?

3. Discuss how teenage pregnancy can result in child abuse to the newborn.

4. What birth control measures would you suggest for Bertha during your postpartal teaching?

CRITICAL INQUIRY EXERCISE

1. Prepare a teaching plan for a woman with cerebral palsy that addresses methods for maintaining an adequate rest and activity pattern.

2. Write a short essay about your feelings regarding adolescent pregnancy, women over age 40 who plan pregnancy, and women with drug addiction who become pregnant. What type of nursing care should they receive?

CRITICAL EXPLORATION

Visit a prenatal clinic for women who are mentally retarded. Observe the visit of a woman at each of the levels of retardation. Note the differences and similarities in instructions given regarding activities, rest, and nutritional needs.

■ Practicing for NCLEX

MULTIPLE-CHOICE QUESTIONS

Circle the letter that corresponds to the best answer for each question.

1. Bobby, age 14, is in her fourth month of pregnancy. To help prevent anemia, the nurse would do which of the following?
   A. Tell Bobby she needs to eat balanced meals and snacks so that she will be well nourished.
   B. Instruct Bobby to report black stools, which indicate that she is bleeding internally due to iron intake.
   C. Instruct Bobby regarding the signs of labor before she completes her fifth month of pregnancy.
   D. Tell Bobby if she takes an iron supplement each day she won't have to eat foods like liver.

2. When planning a teaching strategy for the pregnant adolescent, the nurse should do which of the following?
   A. Inform the teen she should consider the needs of her baby first when eating or planning activity.
   B. Omit information related to minor pains of pregnancy to prevent the adolescent from developing hypochondria.
   C. Explain how healthy eating and exercise habits will help the teen look and feel better.
   D. Emphasize the importance of frequent urine and blood testing to ensure that she is drug-free.

3. Bonnie, 16 years old and 7 months pregnant, has been diagnosed with early symptoms of pregnancy-induced hypertension (PIH). Outcome criteria that would be appropriate for Bonnie would include which of the following? Bonnie:
   A. Regularly performs knee–chest exercises three times daily to strengthen her vascular system
   B. Verbalizes a plan for obtaining schoolwork while resting at home until her baby is born
   C. States her intention to watch for pale mucous membranes and note any cravings, which are signs of PIH
   D. Verbalizes her understanding that she is ill and must remain in bed in order to get well

4. Sheila, age 41, is pregnant and has been scheduled for a serum alpha-fetoprotein level test. The nurse would explain which of the following to Sheila?
   A. One purpose of the test is to determine whether a chromosomal defect is present.
   B. An amniocentesis will not provide the fetal serum specimen needed for the test.
   C. Conditions like open spinal cord cannot be diagnosed through this test.
   D. The test must be performed before the 12th week of pregnancy to prevent fetal damage.

5. Your client has a T2 spinal cord injury and is 6 months pregnant. Which of the following information should be included in pregnancy counseling for her?
   A. She will not be able to feel uterine contractions, so she will need to feel her abdomen often during the last months of pregnancy to detect the tightening that occurs with labor.
   B. She should adjust the footrests on her wheelchair so that she maintains her legs with a sharp bend at the knee to relieve the pressure on her abdomen.
   C. Pregnancy will decrease her risk for urinary tract infections since serum corticosteroid levels are increased in pregnancy.
   D. The enlarged uterus will assist her in urinating, so she will not need to use a catheter or perform the Credé method to be sure she empties her bladder.

6. Joan is in her fourth month of pregnancy and confides to the nurse that she is addicted to heroin and uses prostitution to afford her habit. Which response by the nurse would be most appropriate?
   A. Plan to include tests for sexually transmitted diseases in Joan's future prenatal visits.
   B. Prepare Joan for the high possibility that her baby will be born dead because she has taken heroin.
   C. Record on Joan's chart the need to monitor her baby for hyperbilirubinemia, a complication of heroin abuse.
   D. Tell Joan her baby is in no danger because fetal exposure to narcotics actually strengthens the liver and the lungs.

7. During the postpartal period the nurse would implement which of the following measures for the visually impaired woman to facilitate maternal–child well-being?
   A. Instruct the mother to secure a sighted assistant to help her care for her new infant after she is discharged home.
   B. Limit the time the mother has to care for her child during the first few days to prevent frustration and fatigue.
   C. Speak loudly when explaining self-care measures or infant care measures the mother must use with her baby.
   D. Stress the importance of the mother facing the infant when speaking, to establish eye-to-eye contact and develop trust.

8. Tina is a pregnant cocaine user. Which of the following, if undertaken by Tina, would indicate that a teaching plan for her had been effective?
   A. Tina plans to restrict her cocaine use to smoking a pipe during her last months of pregnancy.
   B. Tina decreases cocaine use once she has completed her pregnancy.
   C. Tina stated she will use crack instead of cocaine while she is pregnant.
   D. Tina voiced plans to seek assistance to help her stop using cocaine.

9. Which of the following information would be most important to provide to a pregnant woman who is drug-dependent?
   A. Her fetus may be born drug-dependent and have withdrawal symptoms.
   B. Marijuana can be used to decrease withdrawal symptoms without fetal harm.
   C. Pregnancy will temporarily take away her desire for drugs and alcohol.
   D. Regular cocaine will not cross the placental barrier, but crack cocaine will.

ALTERNATE FORMAT QUESTIONS

Fill in the Blank

Supply the missing term or the information requested.

1. A pregnant adolescent is regarded as an ——— ——— and can make her own health care decisions and sign permission for her own care.
2. In a pregnant adolescent, cephalopelvic disproportion is suggested by ——— ——— ——— at the beginning of labor, a ——— first stage of labor, and poor ——— ———.

Multiple-Answer Multiple Choice

Circle the letter(s) corresponding to the appropriate answers. Select all that apply.

1. When providing care to a 42-year-old pregnant woman, the nurse would be alert for signs and symptoms of which of the following?
   A. Hypertension of pregnancy
   B. Preterm birth
   C. Post-term birth
   D. Rapid labor
   E. Postpartum hemorrhage

UNIT IV

The Nursing Role in Caring for the Family During Labor and Birth

CHAPTER 18

The Labor Process

CHAPTER OVERVIEW

Chapter 18 provides an overview of the components and process of labor and discusses nursing care of the woman in labor. Problems and concerns that may manifest during each stage of labor are reviewed. The use of the nursing process to plan and provide care throughout the stages of labor is explored.

LEARNING OBJECTIVES

After mastering the content in this chapter, you should be able to do the following:

1. Describe the common theories explaining the onset and progress of labor.
2. Discuss the role of the components of labor: passenger, passage, powers, and psychological impact.
3. Assess a woman in labor, identifying the stage and progression.
4. Formulate nursing diagnoses related to the physiologic and psychological aspects of labor.
5. Establish expected outcomes to meet the needs of the woman and her family throughout the labor process.
6. Implement nursing care for the family during labor.
7. Evaluate outcomes for achievement and effectiveness of nursing care.
8. Identify National Health Goals related to a safe labor and birth that nurses can be instrumental in helping the nation to achieve.
9. Identify areas related to labor and birth that could benefit from additional nursing research or application of evidence-based practice.
10. Use critical thinking to analyze the effectiveness of nursing care measures in meeting the needs of women in labor and their families.
11. Integrate knowledge of nursing care in labor with the nursing process to achieve quality maternal and child health nursing care.

KEY TERMS

amnioinfusion
attitude
breech presentation
cardinal movements of labor
cephalic presentation
crowning
dilatation
effacement
engagement
episiotomy
fetal descent
Leopold's maneuver
lie
lightening
molding
passage
passenger
pathologic retraction ring
physiologic retraction ring
position
powers
ripening
station
transition

■ Mastering the Information

MATCHING

Match the terms or description in Column I with a definition, related statement, or term from Column II. Place the letter corresponding to the answer in the space provided.

COLUMN I

1. ____Attitude
2. ____Crowning
3. ____Amnioinfusion
4. ____Effacement
5. ____Engagement
6. ____Fontanelle
7. ____Labor
8. ____Molding
9. ____Physiologic retraction ring
10. ____Power
11. ____Braxton Hicks

COLUMN II

a. Occurs when the presenting part of the fetus has settled into the pelvis at the level of the ischial spines
b. The shortening and thinning of the cervical canal
c. Membrane-covered spaces at the junction of the main suture lines
d. The degree of flexion the fetus assumes or the relation of the fetal parts to each other
e. The change in shape of the fetal skull produced by the force of the uterine contractions pressing the vertex against the closed cervix
f. A series of events by which uterine contractions expel the fetus and placenta from the woman's body
g. A ridge of the inner uterine surface representing the boundary between the thick active and thinner inactive portions of the uterus
h. The addition of a sterile fluid into the pregnant uterus
i. Irregular uterine cramps, which may signal the impending onset of true labor
j. Supplied by the fundus of the uterus and supplemented by abdominal muscles; results in the expulsion of the fetus from the uterus
k. The appearance of the presenting part of the fetus at the opening in the vagina

Additional Matching Exercises

COLUMN I

1. _____The occiput of the fetus points to the left anterior quadrant in a vertex position.
2. _____The triangular fontanelle points toward the right anterior pelvic quadrant.
3. _____The fetal anus of a breech presentation is pointed toward the right maternal pelvis.
4. _____The fetal chin is facing left across the pelvic midsection.
5. _____The fetal shoulder is located in the right lower posterior pelvic area.

COLUMN II

a. Right scapuloposterior (RAP)
b. Left occipitotransverse (LOT)
c. Left mentotransverse (LMT)
d. Right occipitoanterior (ROA)
e. Left occipitoanterior (LOA)
f. Right sacroanterior (RSaA)

SHORT ANSWER

Supply the missing term or the information requested.

1. Following rupture of the membranes, ______ should be taken every 2 hours because of the possibility of infection.
2. During the process of labor the fetus passes from the ______ through the ______ and ______ to the ______ ______.
3. Three of the six signs of impending labor are ______, ______, and ______.
4. The four integrated concepts contributing to the success of labor include ______(fetus), ______ (woman's pelvis), ______(uterine factors), and ______ (woman's feelings).
5. The four methods by which the fetal position, presentation, and lie are established are combined abdominal ______ and ______, ______ ______, auscultation of ______ ______ ______, and ______.
6. Discuss three of the factors that may influence the beginning of labor.
7. Discuss the role of diaphoresis in temperature regulation during labor.
8. Describe the resulting effect when a body part other than the vertex presents.
9. Describe the process and purpose of Leopold's maneuvers.
10. Discuss the psychological responses of a woman to labor and the nurse's role.
11. Compare and contrast the changes occurring in the maternal pulse and blood pressure with changes occurring in the fetal pulse and blood pressure during contractions.
12. Discuss the role that the father or a significant other might play in the labor experience.
13. Indicate the significance of each of the following abnormal fetal heart rate patterns: fetal tachycardia, fetal bradycardia, late deceleration, variable pattern, sinusoidal pattern.

■ Applying Your Knowledge

CASE STUDY

Effie is a 21-year-old primipara who has completed natural childbirth classes with her coach, her husband. She is admitted at noon to the birthing room after 3 hours of active labor at home. She is dilated 3 cm and 80% effaced. Her sister is with her, and she is concerned about causing her husband to miss time at work needlessly early. He is a low-paid hourly worker, and they are a one-income family.

1. What would you explain to Effie about the progression of her labor, and how would you advise her regarding contacting her husband?
2. How could you support Effie, or teach the family to support Effie, if her husband was not present during the second state of her labor?
3. If labor failed to progress, what additional types of support might Effie need? How might these supports differ for a woman who had had a prior delivery by cesarean birth?
4. How would your support for Effie differ if she were a woman who had previously had a difficult delivery?

CRITICAL INQUIRY EXERCISE

1. Prepare a teaching plan for a woman in labor that addresses methods for maintaining a maximum state of comfort during the first and second stages of labor.

2. Briefly explain how you would support a woman who has decided to put her baby up for adoption through the labor process. How would your support measures differ, if at all, for an adolescent girl?

CRITICAL EXPLORATION

Chart the progression of a woman in the active phases of labor on commercial graph forms or using square-ruled graph paper. Note if the progression appears normal or abnormal by comparison with the chart presented in your text.

■ Practicing for NCLEX

MULTIPLE-CHOICE QUESTIONS

Circle the letter that corresponds to the best answer for each question.

1. Bobby has been experiencing regular, coordinated contractions with cervical dilation moving from 4 cm to 6 cm in the last half-hour, and her membranes are still intact. Bobby is in which stage of labor?
   A. Latent phase of the second stage of labor
   B. Active phase of the first stage of labor
   C. Placental stage or the third stage of labor
   D. Second stage of labor
2. When planning comfort measures to help the woman in active labor tolerate her pain, the nurse must consider which of the following?
   A. Early labor contractions are usually regular, coordinated, and very painful.
   B. If women are properly prepared, they will require no medication to manage their pain.
   C. Pain medication given during the latent phase of labor is not likely to impair contractions.
   D. The active phase of labor can be a time of true discomfort and high anxiety.
3. Sheila is in her first stage of labor and the nurse notices a prominent and observable abdominal indentation that she recognizes as a pathologic retraction ring. The nurse should respond to these findings by doing which of the following?
   A. Inform Sheila that this indentation is normal, to decrease her anxiety.
   B. Instruct Sheila to lie on her right side to prevent pressure on her abdomen.
   C. Recognize this as an indication that labor is almost complete.
   D. Report this danger sign to the physician immediately.
4. Frances is admitted in active labor. The nurse locates fetal heart sounds in the upper left quadrant of her abdomen. The nurse would recognize which of the following?
   A. Frances will probably deliver very quickly and without problems.
   B. This indicates that the fetus is probably in the breech position.
   C. The fetus is in the most common anterior fetal position.
   D. This position is referred to as left anteriopelvic.

5. While interviewing a woman in labor, which information would be least important to obtain?
   A. Whether the pregnancy was planned
   B. The use of drugs or medications during pregnancy
   C. Maternal concerns regarding fetal health
   D. If the woman's mother has come with her

6. When timing the length of a contraction, the nurse would do which of the following?
   A. Ask the woman when the beginning of the contraction is felt, then time the interval from this point until the woman states the contraction has subsided.
   B. Gently palpate the abdomen for the beginning of the tightening of the uterus; time the interval from this point until the uterine tightening subsides.
   C. Lightly touch the abdomen and time the interval from the beginning of the uterine tensing to the beginning of the next tensing.
   D. Note the upward slopes of the contraction on the monitor graph and measure from one upward slope to the next upward slope.

7. Which of the following is very important when performing fetal monitoring?
   A. Informing the mother and significant others that the fetal heart rate will vary during the labor process
   B. Instructing the mother that she must lie supine to obtain the most accurate readings of fetal status
   C. Keeping the monitor strap on the woman's abdomen tightly and securely fitted despite maternal discomfort
   D. Maintaining a continuous watch on the monitor, since it is the primary source of data on maternal-fetal status

8. When preparing a pregnant client for internal electronic fetal monitoring, which of the following would the nurse need to keep in mind?
   A. There is little restriction on maternal ambulation.
   B. It can be applied before rupture of the membranes.
   C. A clearer printout of the fetal heart rate is provided.
   D. It cannot be initiated if the fetal head is engaged.

9. Which assessment finding would lead the nurse to suspect fetal distress?
   A. Fetal heart rate acceleration occurring with fetal movement
   B. Early decelerations occurring during contractions late in labor
   C. Serial fetal blood pH levels of 7.10 to 7.15
   D. Fetus is positioned in the left occipitoanterior area

10. If variable deceleration is noted on the fetal heart monitor, the nurse should do which of the following?
    A. Limit oral and intravenous fluids to decrease maternal fluid volume and decrease circulatory overload.
    B. Prepare a needle and large syringe so that excess amniotic fluid causing the problem can be removed.
    C. Remove oxygen, if present, and instruct the mother to breathe slowly, since this is a sign of hyperventilation.
    D. Turn the mother to a different position to relieve pressure on the umbilical cord and restore circulation.

11. If a woman will be placing her baby up for adoption, which of the following nursing measures should be implemented during labor?
    A. Avoid discussing the baby during the health history to minimize the woman's anxiety.
    B. Support the woman as needed by accepting the decisions she makes regarding holding the baby.
    C. Protect the woman from visitors and family members who might try to change her mind.
    D. Take the baby away as soon as possible after birth to prevent bonding from occurring.

12. After the third stage of labor the nurse may have which of the following responsibilities?
    A. Administering intramuscular oxytocin to facilitate uterine contractility
    B. Monitoring for blood loss greater than 60 cc, indicative of gross hemorrhage
    C. Noting if the placenta makes a Schultze presentation, which is a sign of a major complication
    D. Pushing down on the relaxed uterus to aid in the removal of the placenta

13. Immediately after episiotomy repair, the nurse would do which of the following?
    A. Cleanse the woman's anal area, then perineum and vulva, to remove any fecal incontinence or vaginal secretions.
    B. Monitor the woman for shaking and chilliness, which may indicate an adverse reaction to medications.
    C. Palpate the uterine fundus for size, consistency, and position, and take vital signs to obtain baseline data.
    D. Remove all coverings except a clean, light hospital gown to prevent the development of postpartal fever.

14. Which of the following outcome criteria would be appropriate for the woman in labor without a support person? The client will:
    A. Reunite with her child's father before labor is complete
    B. Verbalize that she felt supported during the labor process
    C. Indicate that she was comfortable going through labor alone
    D. State the labor process was a smooth, rewarding experience

15. Which of the following signs could indicate maternal distress during labor?
    A. Maternal heart rate of 90 to 100 beats per minute during labor
    B. Uterine contractions less frequent and intense as labor progresses
    C. Reports of feeling the need to have a bowel movement
    D. Contractions lasting for approximately 60 to 90 seconds

ALTERNATE FORMAT QUESTIONS

Fill in the Blank

Supply the requested terms.

1. As the fetal head moves from above to below the level of the ischial spines, the station or degree of engagement moves from ——— to ——— stations.
2. The first division of the first stage of labor is the ———————————————— division.
3. The softening of the cervix, which occurs in preparation for labor, is called ——————————.

Multiple-Answer Multiple Choice

Circle the letter(s) corresponding to the appropriate answer(s). Select all that apply.

1. When teaching a pregnant woman about a vaginal birth after cesarean birth (VBAC), which information would be most appropriate to include?
    A. Instructions regarding the labor process are not needed.
    B. The woman may respond as if this is her first labor experience.
    C. The outcome of VBAC is usually without complications.
    D. Women usually prefer cesarean birth to vaginal delivery.
    E. The woman may need oxytocin to help strengthen uterine contractions

Hot Spot Questions

Indicate the term or phrase that describes the fetal position that occurs during the fetal descent phase that is depicted.

1.

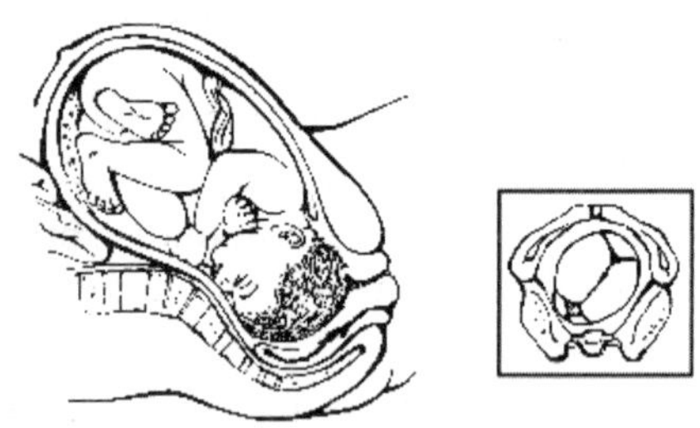

a. Flexion
b. Extension

2.

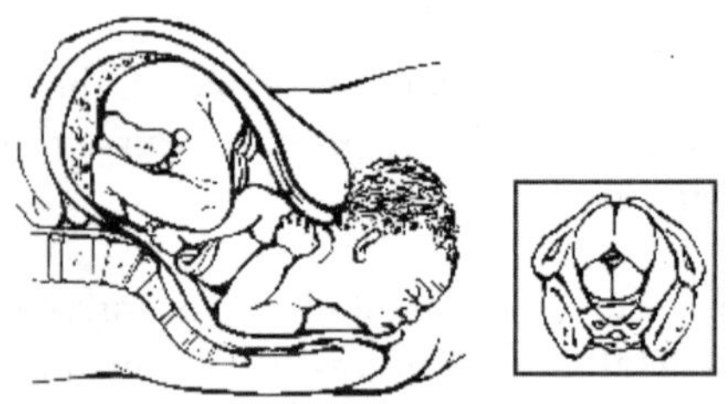

a. Internal rotation
b. Expulsion

CHAPTER 19

Providing Comfort During Labor and Birth

CHAPTER OVERVIEW

Chapter 19 provides an overview of the physiology and perception of pain during labor and principles of pain management, including pharmacologic methods and support of the woman's chosen technique for relaxation and prepared childbirth. The use of the nursing process to plan and provide comfort for the woman throughout labor and delivery is explored.

LEARNING OBJECTIVES

After mastering the content in this chapter, you should be able to do the following:

1. Describe the physiologic basis of contractions during labor and birth and how they relate to theories of pain relief.
2. Identify complementary and alternative therapies that may be used to promote a woman's comfort during labor and birth.
3. Discuss the pharmacologic agents commonly used to provide analgesia and anesthesia during labor and birth.
4. Assess the degree and type of discomfort a woman is experiencing, including her ability to cope with it effectively during labor and birth.
5. Formulate nursing diagnoses related to the effect of pain during labor and birth.
6. Establish expected outcomes to meet the needs of the woman experiencing discomfort during labor and birth.
7. Plan nursing interventions to promote comfort during labor and birth.
8. Implement common complementary and pharmacologic measures for pain relief during labor and birth.
9. Evaluate expected outcomes for effectiveness of nursing care and achievement of a satisfying labor experience for the woman and her family.
10. Identify National Health Goals related to analgesia and anesthesia that childbirth nurses can help the nation achieve.
11. Identify areas related to promoting comfort during labor that could benefit from additional nursing research or application of evidence-based practice.
12. Use critical thinking to analyze ways to maintain family-centered care when analgesia and anesthesia are used in childbirth.
13. Integrate knowledge of pain relief measures during labor and birth with the nursing process to achieve quality maternal and child health nursing care.

KEY TERMS

analgesia
anesthesia
doula
endorphins
epidural anesthesia
pain
pressure anesthesia
pudendal nerve block
transcutaneous electrical nerve stimulation (TENS)

■ Mastering the Information

MATCHING

Match the terms in column I with a definition, example, or related statement from Column II. Place the letter corresponding to the answer in the space provided.

COLUMN I

1. ____Aspiration
2. ____Endorphin
3. ____Spinal anesthesia
4. ____General anesthesia
5. ____Pain
6. ____Meperidine hydrochloride (Demerol)
7. ____Pudendal nerve block
8. ____Regional anesthesia

9. ____Transcutaneous electrical nerve stimulation (TENS)

10. ____Intrathecal narcotics

COLUMN II

a. Injection of anesthetic at the level of the ischial spine; allows for low forceps delivery and episiotomy repair

b. A synthetic narcotic with sedative and antispasmodic action

c. Opiate-like substance produced naturally by the body to reduce pain

d. Minimal fetal effects when compared with systemic anesthetics; leaves the uterus capable of optimal postpartal contraction

e. A subjective symptom; any sensation of discomfort

f. Blockage of afferent fibers, preventing pain from traveling to the spinal cord synapses from the uterus; also effective with extreme back pain

g. A local anesthetic agent injected into the third lumbar space

h. An injection of medication into the spinal canal by way of a catheter

i. Inhalation of vomitus that may cause occlusion of the airway

j. Not a preferred method of pain control in childbirth; requires maternal intubation and increases the risk of aspiration

SHORT ANSWER

Supply the missing term or the information requested.

1. When using pain control drugs during labor and delivery, the risks of fetal bradycardia and maternal hypotension must be weighed against the alternative risk to the mother, which would be ________ ________ ________ ________.

2. Nurses can help the nation meet the goals of reducing maternal and fetal deaths related to analgesia and anesthesia administered during labor and birth by ________, ________, and ________.

3. During uterine contractions of labor, the two major sources of pain are ________ and ________.

4. During the first stage of labor, pain relief must either be ________ or block the synapse sites at spinal column level ________ through ________.

5. Discuss the significance of informing a woman about the use of drugs and the ultimate effect of the various pain relief measures.

6. Explain how knowledge regarding the labor and delivery process might have an impact on the pain experienced during labor.

7. Discuss the importance of timing in the administration of pain relief medications during labor.

8. Discuss the role that a significant other might play in facilitating pain relief during the labor experience.

■ Applying Your Knowledge

CASE STUDY

Alice and Mike are in the birthing room performing breathing exercises during her third hour of true labor. This is their first pregnancy and birth. Alice is dilated 4 cm. Mike appears nervous but is enthusiastic and caring in his coaching.

1. What impact could Mike's nervousness have on Alice and the progress of her labor? What nursing actions would be indicated to address his nervousness?

2. Alice has asked about the risks of using a narcotic analgesic to relieve her pain now. What information would you give her regarding the benefits and disadvantages of analgesic agents at this stage in her labor?

3. What information would you give Alice and Mike about pain control during the second and third phases of labor?

CRITICAL INQUIRY EXERCISE

1. Prepare a pain management plan for a woman in labor that includes two nonpharmacologic pain relief measures and two medical pain relief methods, with nursing implications for monitoring and prevention of drug-related complications.

2. Prepare a checklist of the priority assessments and related nursing actions for managing pain in each stage of labor.

CRITICAL EXPLORATION

Monitor a woman through the entire labor process. Note the methods used by the woman and the health care team to maintain a maximum state of comfort during the first and second stages of labor.

■ Practicing for NCLEX

MULTIPLE-CHOICE QUESTIONS

Circle the letter that corresponds to the best answer for each question.

1. Barbara, a primipara, has been experiencing regular contractions with cervical dilation at 2 cm. Barbara could use which of the following pain relief measures safely?
   A. Acetylsalicylic acid
   B. Breathing exercises
   C. Narcotic analgesic
   D. Pressure anesthesia

2. When planning comfort measures to help the woman in active labor cope with her pain, the nurse must consider which of the following?
   A. Early labor contractions are usually regular, coordinated, and very painful.
   B. If women are properly prepared, they are more likely to require less medication to manage their pain.
   C. Pain medication given during the latent phase of labor is not likely to impair contractions.
   D. The transition phase of labor represents a time of minimum pain and discomfort.

3. Which of the following actions should the nurse take when administering meperidine (Demerol) to a woman in labor?
   A. Administer a dose of naloxone (Narcan) with the medication to boost the antianxiety effects.
   B. Inject the medication into the woman's subcutaneous tissue.
   C. Monitor the newborn for sedation for 3 to 4 hours after the drug is administered.
   D. Reassure the woman that this drug does not cross the placenta.

4. Which of the following would be most helpful for a pregnant woman in labor who has known heart disease?
   A. An epidural block
   B. General anesthesia
   C. Narcotic analgesics
   D. Patient-controlled analgesia

5. Which of the following measures could a nurse take to facilitate comfort in the labor process?
   A. Apply a sanitary pad to decrease discomfort from vaginal secretions.
   B. If membranes are ruptured and the fetus is not engaged, encourage ambulation around the room.
   C. Smooth the wrinkles from bed linen and remove sticky bedclothes.
   D. Tell the woman to remain as still as possible throughout the labor process to decrease stimulation.

ALTERNATE FORMAT QUESTIONS

Multiple-Answer Multiple Choice

Circle the letter(s) corresponding to the appropriate answer(s). Select all that apply.

1. Circle the letter(s) of the drug types listed that are likely to produce a fetal effect. Select all that apply.
   A. Drugs with a molecular weight above 1,000
   B. Drugs with a molecular weight below 600
   C. Drugs that strongly bind to protein
   D. Fat-soluble drugs
   E. Drugs administered to a woman with a premature fetus
   F. Drugs that cause systemic maternal hypotension

2. Circle the letter(s) corresponding with the outcomes that indicate that pain management during labor has been effective. Select all that apply.
   A. The woman's pain is reduced from a level 8 to a level 1.
   B. The fetal heart rate is reduced from 160 to 110.
   C. The woman reports being more relaxed.
   D. The contractions decrease in frequency and become less intense.
   E. The woman's blood pressure is reduced from 130/76 to 100/40.
   F. The woman's pushing efforts are increased.

CHAPTER 20

Cesarean Birth

CHAPTER OVERVIEW

Interruptions in the predictable laboring process and the mechanics of delivery may require a woman to be prepared to deliver her infant by cesarean birth. This chapter reviews both scheduled and emergency cesarean births and examines the pre- and postoperative principles of nursing for the client undergoing a cesarean birth. Reasons for cesarean birth, the surgical procedure, and physiological and psychological responses of the woman are discussed.

LEARNING OBJECTIVES

After mastering the content in this chapter, you should be able to do the following:

1. Describe the indications for cesarean birth.
2. Assess a woman scheduled for cesarean birth for preoperative, intraoperative, and postoperative needs.
3. Formulate nursing diagnoses related to cesarean birth.
4. Establish outcomes that meet the needs of a woman requiring a cesarean birth.
5. Plan appropriate nursing care to ensure family-centered care.
6. Implement common preoperative and postoperative care measures for cesarean birth.
7. Evaluate outcomes for achievement and effectiveness of nursing care.
8. Identify National Health Goals related to cesarean birth that nurses can be instrumental in helping the nation to achieve.
9. Identify areas related to cesarean birth that could benefit from additional nursing research or application of evidence-based practice.
10. Use critical thinking to analyze common complications of cesarean birth to develop preventive strategies.
11. Integrate knowledge of cesarean birth with the nursing process to achieve quality maternal and child health nursing care.

KEY TERMS

cesarean birth
classic cesarean incision
dehiscence
low segment incision
retractors

■ Mastering the Information

Match the terms in Column I with a definition, example, or related statement from Column II. Place the letter corresponding to the answer in the space provided.

COLUMN I

1. _____Transcutaneous electrical nerve stimulation (TENS)
2. _____Patient-controlled analgesia (PCA)
3. _____Stress response
4. _____Epidural analgesia

COLUMN II

a. May result in intense itching and nausea and vomiting
b. Involves applying electrodes to the surface of the skin to effectively control pain by blocking the ability of the cerebral cortex to interpret the incoming sensation
c. Requires self-administration of intravenous narcotic analgesia
d. Results in the release of epinephrine and norepinephrine from the adrenal gland medulla

TRUE OR FALSE

Indicate if the following statements are true or false by placing a "T" or "F" in the space provided.

_____1. Obesity may predispose the skin line repair of a woman who had a cesarean birth to dehiscence.

_____2. Unlike the cesarean birth client who has received general anesthesia, the cesarean birth client who has received an epidural is not at risk for intestinal paralysis.

_____3. The woman who received epidural anesthesia for cesarean birth is limited to a supine position immediately after the procedure.

_____4. Lochia should not be visible for assessment if the woman has a cesarean birth.

SHORT ANSWER

Supply the missing term or the information requested.

1. Why is it a good nursing action to include the expectant woman's support person when giving anticipatory guidance?

2. Why is a sonogram useful to the physician prior to making the incision for a cesarean procedure?

3. Explain why it is of utmost importance that the surgical client be assessed for urinary output following surgery.

4. Identify and discuss three potential maladaptations that may occur in a woman following a cesarean birth procedure if her pain is not controlled.

5. Identify and discuss two supportive pain control methods that can be used to assist the postpartal surgical client. Explain the essential components of these devices.

■ Applying Your Knowledge

CASE STUDY

Lorraine Murphy has delivered her first child under general anesthesia by the cesarean method. The nurse will need to monitor her closely for postpartal and postsurgical complications.

1. What position should Ms. Murphy be placed in when she is brought to the recovery room? Specify how you may help the patient maintain this position.

2. Explain why Ms. Murphy would be in jeopardy for an imbalance of fluid and electrolytes. What important vital signs may alert you to this problem? What drug might be ordered by the physician to ensure uterine contractions?

3. Ms. Murphy has begun to wake up; her words are barely audible, but she manages to ask you for something to drink. How would you respond?

CRITICAL INQUIRY EXERCISE

1. Formulate a nursing care plan that will focus on alleviating fears for the client and family awaiting a cesarean delivery.

2. Compare the pre- and postoperative nursing care needed for the client who delivers vaginally with the client who has undergone a cesarean section delivery.

CRITICAL EXPLORATION

Formulate a teaching plan for a pregnant woman whom you will care for when assigned to the women's health unit. The plan should indicate that this patient has been scheduled for a preplanned surgical procedure. Identify those teaching advantages from your text that you propose will enable the nurse to prepare the patient more efficiently due to the nature of the birthing method. After you have been assigned to the patient on the floor, compare and contrast the teaching points that you selected from your text with those listed in the teaching care plan on the patient's chart.

■ Practicing for NCLEX

MULTIPLE-CHOICE QUESTIONS

Circle the letter that corresponds to the best answer for each question.

1. Mrs. Jordan has been admitted on the unit the day prior to a scheduled cesarean birth. Mrs. Jordan is unable to deliver vaginally due to cephalopelvic disproportion. The nurse instructs Mrs. Jordan on deep breathing exercises as part of the preoperative teaching plan. The rationale for this exercise is to:

A. Promote involution of a traumatized uterus
B. Prevent stasis of mucus in the lungs
C. Prevent pulmonary edema
D. Stimulate the diaphragm to contract

2. The nurse administers ranitidine (Zantac) as ordered prior to a planned cesarean birth to:
A. Neutralize urine acidity
B. Promote uterine contractions
C. Delay uterine contractions
D. Decrease gastric secretions

3. The surgeon plans to perform a low segment incision rather than a classic cesarean. The low incision is more advantageous because:
A. It is made horizontally and high on the woman's abdomen.
B. The procedure is faster since the incision is made through the abdomen and uterus at the same time.
C. The likelihood of a postpartal uterine infection is decreased.
D. The procedure is made with a vertical incision to decrease the chances of reopening.

4. Which of the following would lead the nurse to suspect that a woman who has had a cesarean birth is developing peritonitis?
A. Guarded abdomen
B. Elevated temperature
C. Excessive lochia discharge
D. Episode of painful involuntary contractions

5. If oxytocin is ordered postoperatively for the client who has had a cesarean birth, the most important nursing intervention would be to:
A. Monitor the woman's blood pressure
B. Assess for increased lochia discharge
C. Prevent infection at the incision site
D. Implement measures to promote comfort

ALTERNATE FORMAT QUESTIONS

Fill in the Blank

Supply the missing term or the information requested.

1. During a vaginal delivery a woman loses ——— to ——— mL of blood as compared to a cesarean birth, where she loses ——— to ——— mL.

Multiple-Answer Multiple Choice

Circle the letter(s) corresponding to the appropriate answer(s). Select all that apply.

1. A woman has undergone a cesarean birth is to be discharged. The nurse would instruct the woman to notify her health care provider if she develops which of the following?
A. Burning on urination
B. Drainage at her incision line
C. Decrease in lochia
D. Fever over 100.4° F (38° C)
E. Constipation

CHAPTER 21

The Woman Who Develops a Complication During Labor and Birth

CHAPTER OVERVIEW

Chapter 21 describes and summarizes the more common complications that occur during labor and birth. Women who are most at risk are discussed. The chapter also explores the planning and implementation of care for high-risk women in labor. Common treatments are explained and illustrated. Nursing diagnoses and related intervention skills are emphasized.

LEARNING OBJECTIVES

After mastering the content in this chapter, you should be able to do the following:

1. Define the terms "dystocia" and "dysfunctional labor."
2. Describe the common deviations in the power (force of labor), the passage, or passenger that can cause dystocia or dysfunctional labor.
3. Assess the woman in labor and during birth for deviations from the normal labor process.
4. Formulate nursing diagnoses related to deviations from the normal labor process.
5. Identify appropriate outcomes associated with deviations in normal labor and birth and resultant complications.
6. Plan nursing interventions that will help the family meet established outcomes.
7. Implement care related to potential complications in labor or birth.
8. Evaluate outcomes for achievement and effectiveness of care.
9. Identify National Health Goals related to complications of labor that nurses could be instrumental in helping the nation achieve.
10. Identify areas related to complications of labor that could benefit from additional nursing research or application of evidence-based practice.
11. Use critical thinking to analyze ways to maintain family-centered nursing care when deviations from the normal in labor and birth occur.
12. Integrate the knowledge of deviations from normal in labor and birth with the nursing process to achieve quality maternal and child health nursing care.

KEY TERMS

amniotic fluid embolism
augmentation of labor
battledore placenta
cephalopelvic disproportion
constriction ring
dysfunctional labor
dystocia
external cephalic version
forceps birth
hypertonic uterine contractions
hypotonic uterine contractions
induction of labor
oxytocin
pathologic retraction ring
placenta accreta
placenta circumvallata
placenta marginata
placenta succenturiata
precipitate labor
umbilical cord prolapse
uterine inversion
vacuum extraction

■ Mastering the Information

MATCHING

Match the terms in Column I with a definition, example, or related statement from Column II. Place the letter corresponding to the answer in the space provided.

COLUMN I

1. ____Cephalopelvic disproportion
2. ____Cervical ripening
3. ____Oxytocin
4. ____Dystocia

5. ____McRobert's maneuver
6. ____Pathologic retraction ring
7. ____Vacuum extraction
8. ____Uterine inversion
9. ____Piper forceps
10. ____External cephalic version

COLUMN II

a. Method that is advantageous over forceps births
b. Method used to deliver the head in a breech presentation
c. Ridge across abdomen that signals possible uterine rupture
d. Turning of the uterus inside-out
e. Drug used to induce or augment labor
f. Gentle external pressure used to rotate the position of the fetus
g. Measure involving sharp flexion of woman's thighs onto the abdomen
h. Fetal head too large for passage; small pelvis
i. Change in consistency from firm to soft
j. Sluggishness of contractions or force of labor

STAGES OF LABOR

Indicate whether the following dysfunctions occur in the first (A) or second (B) stage of labor by placing an "A" or "B" in the space provided.

1. —— Protracted active phase
2. —— Prolonged deceleration phase
3. —— Arrest of descent
4. —— Prolonged descent
5. —— Secondary arrest of dilation
6. —— Prolonged latent phase

SHORT ANSWER

Supply the missing term or the information requested.

1. A——— ——— ——— is a warning sign of severe dysfunctional labor and may signal an impending ——— of the uterus.
2. Umbilical cords that have only two vessels are associated with congenital anomalies of the ——— and ——— .
3. Management of a prolapsed cord is aimed toward relieving ——— ———, which will relieve fetal ——— / ———.
4. List and define the three main components of labor.
5. What is one of the major assessments used to detect deviations from normal labor and birth?
6. List three types of abnormal uterine contractions.
7. Name the dysfunctional labor patterns for the first stage of labor.
8. Name three common health problems associated with multiple gestation deliveries.
9. List two dangers of a breech delivery.
10. List four types of abnormal presentation.
11. Name three indications for a forceps delivery.
12. List the two types of breech presentation.

■ Applying Your Knowledge

CASE STUDY

Mrs. Price, age 36, is in premature labor, expecting twins. She is at 36 weeks' gestation, and one of the twins is a breech presentation. This is Mrs. Price's second multiple birth. Her previous delivery of twins resulted in the death of twin A; twin B survived and was later diagnosed with cerebral palsy.

1. What concerns might Mr. and Mrs. Price voice about the impending cesarean section?
2. How should the nurse prepare to respond to their questions and their anxiety?
3. While preparing Mrs. Price for the cesarean section, what changes and vital signs might you assess that would indicate the development of additional problems or complications?
4. Explain why Mrs. Price is at risk for an alteration in fluid and electrolyte balance.

CRITICAL INQUIRY EXERCISE

1. Choose a potential health problem as a complication of labor and write a care plan for this high-risk patient.

2. Formulate a nursing care plan for a woman who is pregnant with her first child and is in prolonged labor.

CRITICAL EXPLORATION

Arrange to visit the labor and delivery care areas in your hospital. Seek assistance from the staff to accompany and monitor a patient who would need surgery after her labor has failed to progress.

■ Practicing for NCLEX

MULTIPLE-CHOICE QUESTIONS

Circle the letter that corresponds to the best answer for each question.

1. Labor may be induced in which of the following women? A woman with:
   A. A fetus in transverse lie
   B. Presenting part engaged
   C. A premature fetus
   D. Cephalopelvic disproportion

2. Standard care plans for a woman in normal active labor include:
   A. Explanation of all procedures being performed
   B. Assessment to determine that the resting tone of the uterus is maintained above 15 mm Hg
   C. Use of sedation whenever requested
   D. Preparing for administration of Pitocin (oxytocin) and use of high forceps

3. A multiparous woman arrived 2 hours ago in active labor with 4 cm of cervical dilation. Now she states that she has a strong urge to push. Which answer most likely describes what is occurring?
   A. She may have cephalopelvic disproportion.
   B. She may need an analgesic or sedation.
   C. She is having a precipitous delivery.
   D. She is having a breech birth.

4. Which of the following would lead the nurse to suspect that a pregnant client has developed an amniotic fluid embolism?
   A. Report of sudden severe chest pain and dyspnea
   B. Evidence of hypotonic contractions and poor force of labor
   C. Report of back pain when ambulating or lying in bed
   D. Rapid cervical dilation of 5 cm/hour

5. To assess a laboring client for ineffective uterine force, the nurse would:
   A. Check the electrolyte panel for the level of carbon dioxide
   B. Obtain a specimen of amniotic fluid and assess for glucose
   C. Monitor contraction duration, strength, and resting tone
   D. Watch the client for elevated respiratory rates during contractions

6. A woman with a fetus in occipitoposterior position would commonly demonstrate which of the following?
   A. Precipitate labor
   B. Acute chest pain
   C. Increased energy levels
   D. Intense back pressure<

ALTERNATE FORMAT QUESTIONS

Fill in the Blank

Supply the missing term or the information requested.

1. ________ ________ causes a marked caput on the newborn's head when used.
2. Immediate management of umbilical cord prolapse is to place the patient in a ______-______ position or ____________________ position.
3. ________ and ________ labor are terms used to describe sluggish contractions.

Multiple-Answer Multiple Choice

Circle the letter(s) corresponding to the appropriate answer(s). Select all that apply.

1. Which conditions place a pregnant woman at high risk for a prolapsed cord?
   A. Premature rupture of membranes
   B. Cephalic fetal presentation
   C. Placenta previa
   D. Intrauterine tumors preventing the presenting part from engaging
   E. A large fetus
   F. Cephalopelvic disproportion preventing firm engagement
   G. Hydramnios
   H. Multiple gestation

2. Name conditions that may place the patient at high risk for uterine rupture during the birthing process.
   A. Premature labor
   B. Abnormal presentation
   C. Multiple gestation
   D. Decreased dosages of oxytocin
   E. Obstructed labor
   F. Traumatic maneuvers of forceps or traction
   G. An episiotomy scar from a previous vaginal birth
   H. Hysterotomy repair tears

3. Identify nontherapeutic effects of oxytocin.
   A. Shorter first stage of labor
   B. Water intoxication due to antidiuresis
   C. Newborn hyperbilirubinemia and jaundice
   D. Tonic uterine contractions with fetal death
   E. Rupture of the uterus

UNIT V

The Nursing Role in Caring for the Family During the Postpartal Period

CHAPTER 22

Nursing Care of the Postpartal Woman and Family

CHAPTER OVERVIEW

Chapter 22 presents an overview of the physiologic and psychological care of the postpartal woman and family. The physiologic changes that occur after childbirth and the emotional effects of childbirth on the entire postpartal family are discussed. The use of the nursing process to plan and provide care for the postpartal family is explored.

LEARNING OBJECTIVES

After mastering the content in this chapter, you should be able to do the following:

1. Describe the psychological and physiologic changes that occur in the postpartal woman.
2. Use the nursing process to determine and address nursing diagnoses related to the physiologic and psychological changes experienced by the woman and her family during the postpartal period.
3. Identify National Health Goals related to the postpartal period that nurses can be instrumental in helping the nation achieve.
4. Use critical thinking to analyze ways that postpartal nursing care can be more family-centered.
5. Synthesize knowledge of the physiologic and psychological changes of the postpartal period using the nursing process to achieve quality maternal and child health nursing care.

KEY TERMS

afterpains
diastasis recti
en face position
engorgement
engrossment
Homans' sign
involution
letting-go phase
lochia alba
lochia rubra
lochia serosa
primary encouragement
sitz bath
taking-hold phase
taking-in phase
uterine atony

■ Mastering the Information

MATCHING

Match the terms in Column I with a definition, example, or related statement from Column II. Place the letter corresponding to the answer in the space provided.

COLUMN I

1. ____Uterine tone assessment
2. ____An empty bladder
3. ____Primary engorgement
4. ____Hydronephrosis
5. ____2,200 to 2,300 kcal, high-protein diet
6. ____Early ambulation
7. ____Sitz bath
8. ____Immediate maternal-child contact
9. ____Oral contraception
10. ____Follow-up examination visit

COLUMN II

a. Measure necessary to promote tissue healing
b. Intervention that reduces risk of perineal infection and promotes comfort
c. A feeling of tenseness of breast tissue on day 3 or 4 postpartum
d. An increase in size of the ureters occurring during pregnancy
e. Activity that can be resumed possibly 2 to 3 weeks postpartum
f. Measure important for detecting potential for postpartum hemorrhage
g. Activity occurring 4 to 6 weeks after delivery
h. Measure to decrease constipation and urinary retention

i. Measure that prevents uterine displacement and promotes accurate assessment of uterine tone
j. Measure important to facilitate bonding

COLUMN I

1. _____Thrombophlebitis
2. _____Urinary retention
3. _____Mastitis
4. _____Hemorrhage

COLUMN II

A. Inflammation of the lining of the blood vessel
B. Major danger during the immediate postoperative period
C. Urine residual greater than 100 cc after catheterization
D. Infection of the breast

SHORT ANSWER

Supply the missing term or the information requested.

1. What is the term describing a time of reflection for a postpartal woman in which she is passive and wants to be ministered to?
2. What is the formation of breast milk called?
3. What is the term describing the incision of the perineum made during the second stage of labor?
4. Briefly compare and contrast the taking-in, taking-hold, and letting-go postpartal phases.
5. Explain the use of sitz bath and ice packs in the care of the postpartal woman who had an episiotomy.
6. Describe the physiologic changes that occur in these structures during the postpartal period: fundus, cervix, vagina.

■ Applying Your Knowledge

CASE STUDY

Rena Despande, age 30, has just given birth to her third daughter. Her husband, age 39, states he wanted a boy but is glad both his wife and the baby are healthy. The baby weighed 10 pounds and Rena had to have an episiotomy.

1. What effect might Rena's husband's hopes for a son have on the couple's postpartal adjustments? What nursing actions might be implemented?
2. Rena shows reluctance to touch her perineal area and resists discussing perineal care. What factors (including culture) might contribute to Rena's discomfort with performing and discussing perineal care?

CRITICAL INQUIRY EXERCISE

1. Write a teaching plan that could be used to prepare new parents for the emotional and physiologic changes occurring after childbirth.
2. What suggestions would you make to a woman who states she has "no time" to perform muscle-strengthening exercises because of childcare and home care responsibilities but says she really wants to get back in shape?

CRITICAL EXPLORATION

1. During a pediatric clinical experience, perform postpartal assessments on two women and compare your findings related to the physiologic and psychological status of each.
2. Interview a woman and her spouse (if possible) during the immediate postpartal period. Attempt to identify signs that the following are being experienced: abandonment, disappointment, or postpartal blues.

■ Practicing for NCLEX

MULTIPLE-CHOICE QUESTIONS

Circle the letter that corresponds to the best answer for each question.

1. Mrs. Peters states that her newborn daughter Millie is "so thin" and "has so little hair." The nurse could best help Mrs. Peters by:
   A. Recognizing that Mrs. Peters is feeling jealous and emphasizing that she doesn't have to find fault with the child to make herself feel attractive
   B. Acknowledging Mrs. Peters' statements, explaining that the child will grow a lot during the first months, and then pointing out many of the baby's good features and behaviors
   C. Asking Mrs. Peters if she was thin as a child and discussing the many dangers of being an underweight, malnourished newborn
   D. Discussing postpartal blues with Mrs. Peters and the fact that negative observations and thoughts are common during this time

2. The nurse, in planning to help a woman adjust to her new baby, must consider which of the following?
   A. The mother will require little assistance since parental love is instinctive.
   B. The more difficult the labor process, the stronger the mother's bond with her child.
   C. It may be natural for the mother to be hesitant initially when touching the child.
   D. Holding the child immediately after birth is overwhelming to a new mother and should be avoided.

3. Mrs. Peters has a 4-year-old son at home and is concerned about his reaction to the new baby. The nurse might do which of the following to best assist this postpartal family?
   A. Instruct Mrs. Peters to write her son a letter and include a picture of the new baby.
   B. Encourage Mrs. Peters to have another family member spend a lot of time with her son.
   C. Arrange for the son to visit with Mrs. Peters and the baby as soon as possible.
   D. Discuss the dangers of sibling rivalry with Mrs. Peters and encourage strict discipline.

4. When examining a postpartal woman, the nurse should immediately report:
   A. A fundus that is palpated 2 cm below the umbilicus on the second postpartal day
   B. A fundus that cannot be located by palpation on the ninth postpartal day
   C. A soft, spongy uterine fundus noted during the first hour postpartum
   D. Red, bloody vaginal discharge on the perineal pad on the first day postpartum

5. During the postpartal period the new mother may experience an alteration in urinary elimination related to loss of bladder sensation. Which of the following data would indicate this problem?
   A. A resonant sound noted on percussion of the lower abdominal area
   B. A firm fundus located 1 cm below the umbilicus on the first postpartal day
   C. Complaints of pain at the episiotomy site, particularly after ambulation
   D. Urinary output greater than 1,500 mL during a 24-hour period

6. The nurse could encourage which of the following measures to decrease the sense of abandonment experienced by the woman and her mate during the postpartal period?
   A. The couple should plan extensive time with the new baby to increase their sense of bonding and decrease jealousy.
   B. The father should be encouraged to share in the care and feeding of the child to increase feelings of involvement.
   C. Discussions of parenting should be avoided during the immediate postpartal period to minimize anticipatory resentment.
   D. The mother should be warned that being jealous of the attention her child is receiving is a sign of postpartal psychosis.

7. Which of the following statements related to the client's nutritional status is a common finding or recommended measure during the postpartal period?
   A. Breastfeeding mothers should limit caloric intake to prevent fat-cell buildup in newborns, which could lead to obesity.
   B. Fluid intake is limited for 48 hours due to the high fluid volume retained in the body after delivery.
   C. High intake of meats, fish, chicken, and dairy products should be encouraged to facilitate good tissue repair.
   D. The mother will have little desire for food or fluids for 24 hours due to the gluconeogenesis that occurs postpartum.

8. Which of the following is an appropriate nursing diagnosis for a postpartal mother with an episiotomy during the first 5 days postpartum?
   A. Anxiety related to vaginal scar formation and decreased body image
   B. Imbalanced nutrition: more than body requirements related to increased appetite
   C. Risk for infection related to lochia and decreased perineal skin integrity
   D. Self-care deficit related to poor opportunity for independence

9. The postpartal mother asks the nurse when her body will return to "normal." The nurse should implement a teaching plan about postpartal body changes that includes which of the following information?
   A. A fast heart rate and thready pulse will occasionally be noted and should be expected.
   B. Menstrual flow will return within 6 to 10 weeks after delivery unless the mother is breastfeeding.
   C. Varicosities and vascular blemishes will disappear by the sixth postpartal week.
   D. The weight gained during pregnancy is usually retained regardless of dietary and exercise efforts.

10. Which of the following would be cause for concern if found during a postpartal assessment?
    A. Diaphoresis during the period immediately after delivery
    B. Hair loss over the postpartal period
    C. Pale coloring of the inner conjunctiva
    D. Reports of slight breast tenderness

11. The most appropriate method for assessing the uterine fundus would be to:
    A. Massage the uterus between the thumb and middle finger until firm, then use a ruler to measure location
    B. Palpate the fundus while the woman has a full bladder to facilitate detection of the uterus
    C. Place both hands below the symphysis pubis and push upward until the lower end of the fundus is located
    D. Support the lower segment of the uterus while palpating the fundus to prevent inversion

12. Placing the infant at the breast to breastfeed has what effect on uterine tone?
    A. Breastfeeding stimulates lactation, which increases the formation of clots in the uterus.
    B. Stimulation of the breast causes oxytocin release and decreased tone in the uterine wall.
    C. The pressure of the infant breastfeeding can cause uterine rupture.
    D. Uterine contraction is stimulated by the infant sucking on the breast.

13. Which of the following is the most appropriate outcome criterion for the postpartal mother and family?
    A. Client demonstrates the procedure for self-examination of the breast, the fundus, and perineal area and states her intent to perform these exams.
    B. Client's temperature is 100.4° to 101°F; no redness or discharge of any kind is noted during the first 48 hours after delivery.
    C. Client does not request pain medication for episiotomy pain and tolerates breast discomfort with minimal comment.
    D. Client prepares a menu including low-calorie foods and minimal intake of meats and bread or starchy food products.

14. The nurse is caring for 14-year-old Lisa, who has decided to give her baby up for adoption. Which of the following should the nurse keep in mind?
    A. Lisa would probably keep her baby if she were given encouragement.
    B. After the delivery Lisa may express a desire to keep her baby, or she may want to continue with the adoption.
    C. During the taking-in phase of the puerperium, the nurse should encourage Lisa to reconsider her decision to abandon her baby.
    D. Lisa should not hold, see, or touch her baby after the delivery to decrease her feelings of loss after giving the child away.

15. An appropriate goal for a postpartal client who complains of being exhausted and unable to sleep would be that the client:
    A. Abstains from performing self-care and rests instead
    B. States she feels rested during the postpartal period
    C. Sleeps during the night in order to stay awake all day
    D. Sleeps 8 hours every night after discharge from the hospital

16. Which of the following might lead the nurse to identify the nursing diagnosis of "Situational low self-esteem related to lack of knowledge regarding psychological changes during the postpartal period" for a postpartal client?
    A. She denies that she has feelings of abandonment or fatigue.
    B. She performs grooming and infant care activities.
    C. She states that she will not be jealous of her child any longer.
    D. She verbalizes that she has conflicting feelings.

ALTERNATE FORMAT QUESTIONS

Fill in the Blank

1. ——— exercises consist of contracting and relaxing the muscles of the perineum.
2. The pink or brownish vaginal drainage noted around the fourth postpartal day is called ———.

Multiple-Answer Multiple Choice

Circle the letter(s) corresponding to the appropriate answer(s). Select all that apply.

1. Data supporting a diagnosis of "Risk for deficient fluid volume related to subinvolution" would include:
    A. Blood pressure of 90/62 noted on the third day after delivery
    B. Firm uterine fundus located at standard measurement level
    C. Lochia saturating one perineal pad per hour 12 hours postpartum
    D. Pulse slow and bounding during the first postpartal day
    E. Temperature of 100.0 degrees F (37.8 degrees C) 4 hours postpartum

2. Which of the following nursing interventions would be appropriate when caring for an client with an episiotomy who has the nursing diagnosis "Pain related to perineal sutures"?
    A. Apply ice packs to the perineal incision site to decrease edema.
    B. Encourage the client to contract and relax perineal muscles.
    C. Instruct client to use petroleum jelly or mineral oil on the episiotomy as desired.
    D. Limit pain medication to prevent dependence on narcotic analgesics.
    E. Encourage sexual activity after one week to loosen sutures.

3. What characteristics would indicate that lochia flow is normal?
    A. Lochia amount increases with strenuous exercise.
    B. Lochia contains no large clots.
    C. Lochia is absent during the first 1 to 3 weeks after a cesarean birth.
    D. Lochia is white for the first 1 to 3 days postpartum.
    E. Lochia has the same odor as menstrual blood.

CHAPTER 23

Nursing Care of the Woman and Family Experiencing a Postpartal Complication

CHAPTER OVERVIEW

A woman experiencing a postpartal complication is subject to difficulty in bonding with her child. If the illness responds poorly to treatment, her potential to give birth to another child may be threatened. Many postpartal complications can be prevented with the support of a health team's assessment skills and the ability of each professional caring for the postpartal patient to evaluate findings and intervene appropriately.

LEARNING OBJECTIVES

After mastering the content in this chapter, you should be able to do the following:

1. Describe common deviations from the normal that can occur during the puerperium.
2. Assess a woman and her family for deviations from the normal during the puerperium.
3. Formulate nursing diagnoses related to deviations from the normal during the puerperium.
4. Identify expected outcomes of a postpartal woman experiencing a complication.
5. Plan interventions that meet the special needs of a family with a postpartal complication, such as planning for an extended hospitalization.
6. Implement nursing care when a postpartal complication such as hemorrhage, infection, pregnancy-induced hypertension, or postpartal psychosis develops.
7. Evaluate expected outcomes for achievement and effectiveness of care.
8. Identify National Health Goals related to postpartal complications that nurses can help the nation achieve.
9. Identify areas related to care of women with postpartal complications that could benefit from additional nursing research or application of evidence-based practice.
10. Use critical thinking to analyze ways that promote family-centered nursing care when a postpartal complication occurs.
11. Integrate knowledge of postpartal complications with the nursing process to achieve quality maternal and child health nursing care.

KEY TERMS

endometritis
mastitis
peritonitis
postpartal depression
postpartal psychosis
thrombophlebitis

■ Mastering the Information

MATCHING

Match the terms in Column I with a definition, example, or related statement from Column II. Place the letter corresponding to the answer in the space provided.

COLUMN I

1. _____Thrombophlebitis
2. _____Endometritis
3. _____Perineal hematomas
4. _____Postpartal depression
5. _____Peritonitis
6. _____Urinary retention
7. _____Mastitis

COLUMN II

a. A collection of blood in the subcutaneous layer of the perineum
b. Infection of the breast
c. Result of edema of the bladder from pressures during childbirth
d. Overwhelming sadness extending beyond the immediate postpartum period
e. Inflammation of the lining of a blood vessel with the formation of blood clots
f. Infection of the peritoneal cavity
g. Infection of the lining of the uterus

TRUE OR FALSE

Indicate if the following statements are true or false by placing a "T" or "F" in the space provided.

______1. The majority of the complications occurring during the puerperium are preventable.

______2. Women who experience blood loss greater than 500 cc in 24 hours are traditionally considered to be hemorrhaging and may require blood replacement.

______3. An elevated level of human chorionic gonadotropin (hCG) is present if the postpartal woman has retained placental fragments after the birth of the placenta.

______4. Most postpartal infections are caused by staphylococcal organisms.

SHORT ANSWER

Supply the missing term or the information requested.

1. The four reasons that are most often found to be the precipitating causes of postpartal hemorrhage are ———, ———, ———, and ———.
2. Define disseminated intravascular coagulation (DIC).
3. What are the common causes of DIC during the postpartal period?
4. What is the rationale that supports teaching women to wipe the perineal area from front to back when cleansing or removing feces?
5. Endometritis is a preventable postpartal complication that may lead to a more serious illness. What are the important components of the nurse's assessment to determine the early signs of endometritis?
6. Explain why it is important to inspect the placenta after an uncomplicated delivery.

■ Applying Your Knowledge

CASE STUDY

Mrs. Lawson, age 36, gravida 3 para 3, is suffering from a puerperal infection during the postpartum period. You are assigned to work with Mrs. Lawson on the sixth day of her hospital stay.

1. What would be considered a probable cause of Mrs. Lawson's condition?
2. Are there any measures that could have been considered to avoid this illness?

As you review Mrs. Lawson's records you find that her assessment, several days ago, revealed data that may have suggested the beginning of her present illness.

3. What are some indicators that patients presenting with Mrs. Lawson's illness often exhibit?
4. Discuss the therapeutic measures that will be used to assist this patient.

CRITICAL INQUIRY EXERCISE

1. Prepare a discharge teaching packet for a client with thrombophlebitis.

2. Consider the risk of exposure to an infection during delivery. Develop a set of guidelines that can serve as protective measures against the development of endometritis.

CRITICAL EXPLORATION

Review the policy of the agency where you are doing your maternal health clinical rotation. Identify the ward's policy on the nurse's authority to order blood from the blood bank for a client who is experiencing a postpartal hemorrhage.

■ Practicing for NCLEX

MULTIPLE-CHOICE QUESTIONS

Circle the letter that corresponds to the best answer for each question.

1. Which assessment finding would lead the nurse to suspect a postpartal complication?
   A. Lochia rubra 12 hours after birth
   B. Temperature of 100.4°F or less
   C. Blood loss of more than 12 oz/24 hrs
   D. 20 to 24 sanitary pads saturated/24 hrs

2. Mrs. Jones is experiencing signs of shock about 3 hours after delivery. Which of the symptoms below will the nurse expect to find when assessing Mrs. Jones?
   A. Diastolic blood pressure increased more than 10 mm Hg
   B. Decreased pulse rate
   C. Rapid respirations
   D. Flushed face

3. Which medication would the nurse expect to administer as ordered for a client who is experiencing postpartum hemorrhage from uterine atony?
   A. Apresoline
   B. Zaroxolyn
   C. Methergine
   D. Proventil

4. Which of the following is viewed as a risk factor for a woman developing a postpartal infection?
   A. Thyroid toxicosis
   B. Excessive blood loss
   C. Pregnancy-induced hypertension
   D. Negative Rh factor

5. Which measure would be most appropriate when caring for the client who has experienced a fourth-degree perineal laceration?
   A. Encourage her to douche at least once a week to reduce organisms that may come in contact with the perineal area.
   B. Administer analgesic rectal suppositories to promote comfort.
   C. Encourage fluid intake and foods high in fiber.
   D. Administer an enema when necessary to prevent constipation.

ALTERNATE FORMAT QUESTIONS

Fill in the Blank

Supply the missing term or the information requested.

1. When assessing lochia to detect a cervical tear that occurred during the birthing process, the nurse would note that blood from a cervical tear is ________________ than normal lochia.

2. The nurse would weigh ________ ________ to get an accurate measurement of blood loss from lochia.

Multiple-Answer Multiple Choice

Circle the letter(s) corresponding to the appropriate answer(s). Select all that apply.

1. Identify the cardinal signs of postpartal-induced hypertension.
   A. Elevated blood pressure
   B. Urinary frequency
   C. Edema
   D. Proteinuria
   E. Perspiration

CHAPTER 24

Nursing Care of the Newborn and Family

CHAPTER OVERVIEW

Chapter 24 presents exercises to refine knowledge of newborn assessment and care. It is important that the nurse be able to evaluate findings obtained on assessment and intervene appropriately when these findings suggest underlying pathology. This chapter assists the student in recognizing "normal" findings and differentiating them from abnormal findings. Anticipatory guidance with regard to feeding, daily routines, and the characteristics of stools is addressed.

LEARNING OBJECTIVES

After mastering the content in this chapter, you should be able to do the following:

1. Describe the normal characteristics of a term newborn.
2. Assess a newborn for normal growth and development.
3. Formulate nursing diagnoses related to a newborn and/or family of a newborn.
4. Identify expected outcomes for a newborn and family during the first 4 weeks of life.
5. Plan nursing care to augment normal development of a newborn, such as ways to aid parent–child bonding.
6. Implement nursing care of a normal newborn, such as administering a first bath or instructing parents on how to care for their newborn.
7. Evaluate expected outcomes to determine the effectiveness of nursing care and outcome achievement.
8. Identify National Health Goals related to newborns that nurses could help the nation achieve.
9. Identify areas related to newborn assessment and care that could benefit from additional nursing research or application of evidence-based practice.
10. Use critical thinking to analyze ways that the care of a term newborn can be more family-centered.
11. Integrate knowledge of newborn growth and development and immediate care needs with the nursing process to achieve quality maternal and child health nursing care.

KEY TERMS

acrocyanosis	meconium
caput succedaneum	milia
cavernous hemangioma	mongolian spot
central cyanosis	natal teeth
cephalhematoma	neonatal period
conduction	neonate
convection	nevus flammeus
Crede treatment	physiologic jaundice
erythema toxicum	pseudomenstruation
evaporation	radiation
hemangioma	strawberry hemangioma
jaundice	subconjunctival hemorrhage
kangaroo care	thrush
kernicterus	transitional stool
lanugo	vernix caseosa

■ Mastering the Information

MATCHING

Match the terms in Column I with a definition, example, or related statement from Column II. Place the letter corresponding to the answer in the space provided.

COLUMN I

1. ____Subconjunctival hemorrhage
2. ____Physiologic jaundice
3. ____Crede treatment
4. ____Extrusion reflex
5. ____Nevus flammeus
6. ____Cremasteric reflex
7. ____Strawberry hemangioma
8. ____Brown fat

9. ____Neonatal period
10. ____Natal teeth

COLUMN II

a. A special tissue found in mature newborns to conserve or produce body heat
b. Prophylaxis against gonorrheal conjunctivitis for the newborn
c. Pressure during birth causing a red spot on the sclera
d. Movement upward of the testes when the inner aspect of the thigh is stroked
e. Infant attempting to refuse solid foods
f. Yellowing of the skin as a result of the breakdown of fetal red blood cells
g. Port-wine stain/hemangioma lesion level with skin
h. Vascular tumor of the skin, elevated areas formed by immature capillaries and epithelial cells
i. One or two dental eruptions present at birth
j. Time from birth through the first 28 days

TRUE OR FALSE

Indicate if the following statements are true or false by placing a "T" or "F" in the space provided.

______1. Infants who do not void within 24 hours after birth might have urethral stenosis.

______2. Murmurs heard when examining the neonate usually indicate cardiac anomalies and must be corrected surgically.

______3. An increased number of leukocytes in the newborn's serology test suggests a response to an infection.

______4. A circumcision prevents phimosis and reduces the incidence of urinary tract infections.

SHORT ANSWER

Supply the missing term or the information requested.

1. The average respiratory rate for the neonate is how many breaths per minute?

2. The infant is vulnerable to heat instability and loses heat readily through four separate mechanisms. What are they?

3. List the six criteria described by Brazelton that are used as the basis to evaluate the newborn's behavioral capacity.

4. Describe and contrast the stools of a bottle- and breast-fed infant.

5. Why would the nurse be concerned after learning that a neonate has not passed a stool by 24 hours after birth?

6. Identify the behaviors exhibited by the newborn in the first period of reactivity and in the second period of reactivity.

7. Explain the principles of safety when placing a child in a car seat or using a car seat belt.

8. Discuss the potential adverse effects of elective surgery to the male infant's penis.

9. Explain why parents, visitors, and hospital personnel with cold sores should not care for the newborn infant.

■ Applying Your Knowledge

CASE STUDY

Today Mrs. Calland delivered vaginally a baby boy. He was born at 38 weeks' gestation and weighed 3,200 g. Mrs. Calland plans to breastfeed her baby. You are assigned as the nurse to take care of her and her baby.

1. Shortly after delivery a number of reflexes were tested on the infant. List the reflexes that were tested and explain which maneuvers were used to complete the tests.

2. Within 12 hours after birth the infant passed a sticky black stool. Explain why this should not alarm you.

3. On the day of discharge, baby boy Calland appears to have yellow skin and sclerae. What lab test might be ordered at this time? What would be indicated if the results are higher than normal values?

4. What effect does breastfeeding have on this condition?

CRITICAL INQUIRY EXERCISE

1. Formulate a nursing care plan that will focus on nursing care for a male infant who has difficulty maintaining an appropriate body temperature.

2. Develop a neonatal admission assessment form that might be used in a newborn nursery.

CRITICAL EXPLORATION

1. Identify a mother who has just given birth to her first child. Formulate a teaching plan that will focus on immediate care needs for the newborn in the home environment. Discuss this information with the mother and include the father of the child, if he is available.

2. Locate the resources in your community that help families obtain car seats when they cannot afford to buy one.

3. Identify a newborn infant who is more than 24 hours old. Perform the Brazelton Neonatal Behavioral Assessment and present your findings to the class.

■ Practicing for NCLEX

MULTIPLE-CHOICE QUESTIONS

Circle the letter that corresponds to the best answer for each question.

1. The nurse is performing the morning assessment of baby boy Lee, born yesterday at 39 weeks' gestation and weighing 3,500 g. When assessing the chest compared to the head, the nurse would expect:
   A. The chest circumference to be about 2 cm less than the head circumference
   B. The chest and head circumference to be equal
   C. The head circumference to be about 2 cm less than the chest circumference
   D. The head circumference to be about 3 cm more than the chest circumference

2. A neonate's temperature is slightly subnormal 1 hour after birth. Which action would be most appropriate?
   A. Take the infant to the mother for bonding and transfer of body heat after the mother rests for an hour.
   B. Place a second stockinette on the infant's head.
   C. Administer a warm bath with temperature slightly higher than usual.
   D. Place the infant under a radiant warmer or in a heated isolette.

3. Which assessment finding in a neonate would cause the nurse to notify the physician?
   A. Breast tissue slightly engorged
   B. Heart rate of 170 beats per minute
   C. Crepitus palpated at the clavicular area
   D. Frog-like positioning of the lower extremities

4. When assessing the neonate, which finding would the nurse interpret as a pathological disturbance?
   A. Heart rate of 130 bpm
   B. Rhonchi auscultated over the lung area
   C. Neonate's abdomen, not the chest, rises when breathing
   D. Nonpalpable femoral pulses

5. The nurse attempts to elicit the Moro reflex in a neonate by:
   A. Stroking the cheek near the corner of the mouth
   B. Loudly tapping the bassinet
   C. Placing a substance on the anterior portion of neonate's tongue
   D. Stroking the side of the foot to have the toes fan out

ALTERNATE FORMAT QUESTIONS

Fill in the Blank

Supply the missing term or the information requested.

1. The time of birth through the first 28 days of life is termed the ______________ ______________.
2. The average heart rate for the neonate is ______.

Multiple-Answer Multiple Choice

Circle the letter(s) corresponding to the appropriate answer(s). Select all that apply.

1. Which interventions would be most appropriate to promote parental–newborn bonding?
   A. Let the mother rest for 1 to 2 hours after birth before initiating contact with the newborn.
   B. Leave an amulet or other good-luck charm from the parents in the newborn's bassinet.
   C. Compliment the newborn whose parents are from Cambodia or Laos about their desire to "ward off spirits."
   D. During first period of activity, ask which parent wants to hold the newborn and place him or her in the parent's arms.
   E. Encourage parents to hold and provide care for newborn while still in the hospital.

CHAPTER 25

Nutritional Needs of the Newborn

CHAPTER OVERVIEW

Chapter 25 reviews the nutritional needs of the newborn. The nutrients in breast milk and commercially prepared formulas are evaluated and contrasted. The physiology of good nutrition is important for the growth and development of the newborn infant. After reading this chapter the student should know how to assess and evaluate the mother's ability to feed the infant and the infant's response to nutritional intake. The chapter also enables the student to provide nursing care for the mother and infant using a nursing care plan as a teaching tool.

LEARNING OBJECTIVES

After mastering the content in this chapter, you should be able to do the following:

1. Describe the nutritional requirements of the term newborn.
2. Assess the nutritional intake of a newborn to determine adequate nutritional status.
3. Formulate nursing diagnoses related to newborn nutrition.
4. Identify appropriate outcomes for the newborn and mother related to nutrition.
5. Plan a method of infant feeding with a mother that will be satisfying for both her and the infant.
6. Implement or help parents implement feeding procedures with newborn infants.
7. Evaluate outcomes for achievement and effectiveness of care.
8. Identify National Health Goals related to newborn nutrition that nurses can be instrumental in helping the nation achieve.
9. Identify areas related to nutrition and newborns that could benefit from additional nursing research or application of evidence-based practice.
10. Use critical thinking to assist mothers with nutritional problem solving and making newborn nutrition more family-centered.
11. Integrate the knowledge of normal newborn nutrition with the nursing process to achieve quality maternal and child health nursing care.

KEY TERMS

areola	interferon
bifidus factor	lactiferous sinuses
colostrum	lactoferrin
engorgement	let-down reflex
foremilk	lysozyme
hind milk	prolactin

■ Mastering the Information

MATCHING

Match the terms in Column I with a definition, example, or related statement from Column II. Place the letter corresponding to the answer in the space provided.

COLUMN I

1. ____Adrenocorticosteroid hormone
2. ____Lactose
3. ____Histidine
4. ____Linoleic acid
5. ____Lactiferous sinuses
6. ____Oxytocin
7. ____IgA
8. ____Soap
9. ____Casein
10. ____Colostrum
11. ____Nipple rolling
12. ____Lysozyme
13. ____Hind milk
14. ____Lactoferrin
15. ____Fluoride

COLUMN II

a. Substance that binds large molecules of foreign proteins, including viruses and bacteria; prohibits absorption through the gastrointestinal tract
b. Substance that probably plays a role in assisting mammary glands to secrete milk
c. Hormone of the posterior pituitary gland that aids in uterine contractions
d. Procedure used in preparation for breastfeeding to stimulate the nipple to protrude and remove adhesions
e. An amino acid essential for infant growth found in human breast milk and cow's milk
f. Substance contraindicated when breastfeeding; tends to cause the nipples to dry and crack
g. Thin, watery, yellow fluid consisting of protein, sugar, fat, water, minerals, vitamins, and maternal antibodies
h. Reservoirs for breast milk located behind the nipple
i. The protein in cow's milk
j. Iron-binding protein in breast milk interfering with the growth of pathogenic bacteria
k. Necessary mineral for building sound teeth and resistance to tooth decay
l. An enzyme in breast milk that actively destroys bacteria by dissolving their cell membranes
m. "New milk" formed after the let-down reflex
n. Sugar nutrients found in breast milk that provide ready glucose for rapid brain growth
o. A fatty acid not found in skim milk but is necessary for growth and skin integrity in infants

TRUE OR FALSE

Indicate if the following statements are true or false by placing a "T" or "F" in the space provided.

______ 1. Infants who are fed by propping the bottles are in potential danger of aspirating fluids.

______ 2. Infants put to bed with a bottle of milk risk developing "baby bottle syndrome."

______ 3. If a woman is experiencing sore nipples from breastfeeding, she should use a hand pump to express the milk manually until the nipples have had a chance to heal.

______ 4. Colostrum is the primary constituent of breast milk during the first 3 months of feeding.

______ 5. Oxytocin is released by breastfeeding and stimulates contractions.

______ 6. The more often breasts are emptied, the more efficiently they will fill and continue to maintain a good supply of milk.

______ 7. Placing the breastfed infant over one shoulder and gently stroking his or her back is the best position for burping him or her.

______ 8. Sore nipples are a contraindication for breastfeeding.

SHORT ANSWER

Supply the missing term or the information requested.

1. ______ ______ ______ ______ allows progesterone levels to drop and stimulates the production of the hormone called ______.
2. Prolactin-releasing factor stimulates the ______ ______ gland, which responds with active production of ______.
3. For the woman who might be experiencing preterm labor, nipple rolling is contraindicated because the release of ______ may lead to ______ ______ ______

■ Applying Your Knowledge

CASE STUDY

Ms. Jackson delivered an 8-lb, 6-oz baby girl about 1 hour before your arrival to the clinical site this morning. Your instructor has assigned you to Ms. Jackson for the next 2 days of your clinical rotation. Her prenatal record indicates that she was considering breastfeeding but had not decided at the time of birth. You will need to be prepared to answer her questions about breastfeeding.

1. Compare the advantages and disadvantages of breastfeeding for the infant and mother.
2. What are some appropriate measures to relieve breast engorgement?

3. State how the infant should be properly placed on the breast for feeding.

4. What are some common reasons why breastfed infants do not suck well?

CRITICAL INQUIRY EXERCISE

1. Mrs. Jones' home has its own well. She will be preparing formula for her newborn infant. Outline the steps of sterilization to teach her how to prepare the formula and supplement.

2. Design a teaching tool for parents about the techniques and safeguards of feeding for breast- and bottle-fed babies.

CRITICAL EXPLORATION

1. Survey your community for agencies that promote infant nutrition and parental education. After compiling the list, inform your clients of these agencies before their discharge.

2. Review the nursing care plans in your clinical areas for a mother and infant scheduled for discharge planning at your hospital. Note the information pertinent to infant nutrition. Exercise your teaching skills by providing this information to a parent the day before discharge. On the day of discharge, assess the effectiveness of your teaching by interviewing your client. Create your own evaluation tool.

■ Practicing for NCLEX

MULTIPLE-CHOICE QUESTIONS

Circle the letter that corresponds to the best answer for each question.

1. Jane Albright is breastfeeding her baby girl, whom she delivered at 6 this morning, weighing 6 lb 7.5 oz. The labor and delivery for mother and infant were uneventful. During the first feeding, Mrs. Albright asks how long her baby should suck on each breast per feeding. The nurse's best response would be which of the following?
   A. The infant should start nursing about 15 minutes on each breast.
   B. Five minutes on each breast for each feeding will be sufficient for today.
   C. Nurse only on one breast today for 5 minutes per feeding and start alternating breasts with the first feeding tomorrow.
   D. Ten minutes at each breast will be sufficient and will also keep the infant from becoming fatigued.

2. When counseling a new mother on breastfeeding, the nurse would know that the most important ingredient for success is to:
   A. Teach the client how to relax
   B. Place the infant correctly on the breast
   C. Teach the client about holding the newborn in the various feeding positions
   D. Wait until the newborn actively demands a feeding

3. On the second postpartum day, the nurse observes that a new mother is washing her breast and hands with soap just before she is to receive her infant for the next feeding. The nurse's action, if any, would be governed by which of the following statements?
   A. Good breast hygiene is necessary to avoid the spread of pathogens from the mother's skin to the newborn.
   B. The client should not clean her breast and hands in preparation for feeding until the infant has arrived in the room.
   C. Cleansing the breast with soap may lead to nipple soreness and dryness.
   D. Washing the breasts increases milk production that may be wastefully expressed before the infant is to be fed.

4. On the third postpartum day, Mrs. Jacobs tells the nurse that she sometimes has difficulty getting her daughter to suck. She describes the infant opening her mouth when the breast touches her face but turning her head in the opposite direction. The nurse would explain that this behavior is related to:
   A. The infant's immaturity and unfamiliarity with the technique of feeding
   B. The extrusion reflex, which is normal for newborns; demonstrates the need for much assistance to ensure adequate nutrition
   C. The rooting reflex, which suggests improper technique when placing the infant on the breast
   D. Turning neck reflex, which suggests that breastfed infants are most sensitive to tactile stimulation

5. A new mother reports that her daughter often falls asleep at feedings before she has taken in enough nutrients. Which of the following statements would be a helpful suggestion?
   A. Wash the infant's face with cool water.
   B. Give the infant a bath before alternating breasts to complete the feeding.
   C. Rub the fontanel of the infant's head gently.
   D. Lightly tickle the bottom of the newborn's feet.

6. Which of the following preparations of commercial formulas would the nurse suggest as being the least expensive?
   A. Powder to be combined with water
   B. Condensed liquid to be diluted with equal parts of water
   C. "Ready to pour" type
   D. Individually prepackaged

7. Choose the correct statement to be used to calculate a nutrient needed for the newborn.
   A. Fluid needs are approximately 100 cc/kg body weight/day.
   B. Fat needs are approximately 20 g/kg body weight/day.
   C. Protein needs are 2.2 g/kg body weight/day.
   D. Caloric needs are 100 kcal/kg body weight/day.

ALTERNATE FORMAT QUESTIONS

Fill in the Blank

Supply the missing term or the information requested.

1. ______ milk is produced by the alveolar cells of the __________ gland in the presence of the hormone prolactin.
2. The infant promotes continuous milk production by ______________________________.
3. An infant that is 1.5 months old and weighs 5 kg would require ______ to ______ calories per kilogram of body weight every 24 hours for adequate growth.

Multiple-Answer Multiple Choice

Circle the letter(s) corresponding to the appropriate answer(s). Select all that apply.

1. Which of the following is true about newborn nutrition and nutritional needs?
   A. The caloric requirements in the neonatal period exceed those at any other age.
   B. An infant up to 2 months of age requires 50 to 60 calories per kilogram of body weight (22.7 to 27.3 kcal/lb) every 24 hours.
   C. The caloric requirement at 1 year of age is 100 kcal/kg, or 45 kcal/lb/day.
   D. The 6-month-old has a caloric requirement similar to an adult requirement of 42 kcal/kg, or 20 kcal/lb/day.
   E. The actual caloric requirement of an infant depends on an infant's individual activity level and growth rate.

2. Which of the following is an acceptable guideline for use and storage of canned formula?
   A. The nutrients in canned formula may be enhanced with whole milk.
   B. Spring water in most instances is found to be clean and more suitable in preparing infant formula.
   C. Store the unused portions of the infant's bottle at room temperature after feeding.
   D. Formula in an open can should be used or discarded in 24 hours.
   E. If the microwave is used to warm formula, shake the formula well to mix the cooled and warmed milk.

CHAPTER 26

Nursing Care of the High-Risk Newborn and Family

CHAPTER OVERVIEW

The high-risk neonate may have difficulty establishing respirations at birth, and this newborn will need care from a skilled professional health team. The neonate's problem may be related to gestational age, physiologic complications, pregnancy complications, or unhealthy maternal lifestyle. After completion of this chapter the student will be able to care for the high-risk newborn who needs resuscitation and maintenance of respiration.

LEARNING OBJECTIVES

After mastering the content in this chapter, you should be able to do the following:

1. Define small-for-gestational-age infant, term infant, large-for-gestational-age infant, preterm infant, and postterm infant and describe common illnesses that occur in these and other high-risk newborns.
2. Assess a high-risk newborn to determine if safe transition to extrauterine life has occurred.
3. List nursing diagnoses related to a high-risk newborn.
4. Identify appropriate expected outcomes for a high-risk newborn and family.
5. Plan novice-level nursing care focusing on priorities to stabilize a high-risk newborn's body systems.
6. Implement novice-level nursing care for a high-risk newborn.
7. Evaluate expected outcomes to determine achievement and effectiveness of care.
8. Identify National Health Goals related to high-risk newborns that nurses could be instrumental in helping the nation achieve.
9. Identify areas related to the care of high-risk newborns that could benefit from additional nursing research or application of evidence-based practice.
10. Use critical thinking to analyze the special crisis imposed on families when alterations of newborn development or neonatal illness occur to make nursing family-centered.
11. Integrate knowledge of the needs of a high-risk infant with the nursing process to achieve quality maternal and child health nursing care.

KEY TERMS

apnea
apparent life-threatening event
appropriate for gestational age
brown fat
caudal regression syndrome
cephalopelvic disproportion
developmental care
dysmature
extracorporeal membrane oxygenation (ECMO)
extremely-very-low-birthweight infant
gestational age
hemorrhagic disease of the newborn
hydrops fetalis
hyperbilirubinemia
hyperglycemia
hypocalcemia
hypoglycemia
intrauterine growth retardation
kernicterus
large-for-gestational-age infant
low-birthweight infant
macrosomia
ophthalmia neonatorum
periodic respirations
periventricular leukomalacia
postterm infant
postterm syndrome
preterm infant
primary apnea
retinopathy of prematurity
secondary apnea
shoulder dystocia
small-for-gestational-age infant
term infant
transient tachypnea
very-low-birthweight infant

■ Mastering the Information

MATCHING

Match the terms in Column I with a definition, example, or related statement from Column II. Place the letter corresponding to the answer in the space provided.

COLUMN I

1. _____Term
2. _____Low birthweight
3. _____Postterm
4. _____Small for gestational age
5. _____Large for gestational age

COLUMN II

A. Infant whose weight falls below the 10th percentile of weight for gestational age

B. Infant whose weight falls above the 90th percentile of weight for age

C. Infant weighing less than 2,500 g

D. Infant born after the onset of week 43 of pregnancy

E. Infant born after week 38 or before week 43 of pregnancy

TRUE OR FALSE

Indicate if the following statements are true or false by placing a "T" or "F" in the space provided.

______1. A newborn's attempt to raise his or her body temperature increases his or her need for oxygen.

______2. A newborn's attempt to raise his or her body temperature increases his or her metabolic rate.

______3. Hypercalcemia is a common nutritional problem of the small-for-gestational-age infant.

______4. Infants of drug-dependent mothers become symptomatic approximately 48 hours after birth.

SHORT ANSWER

Supply the missing term or the information requested.

1. Describe the respiratory pattern of primary apnea.
2. Discuss two causes of intrauterine growth retardation and state one example of each.
3. Explain the concept of extracorporeal membrane oxygenation (ECMO).
4. Discuss how periodic respiration differs from true apnea and periodic apnea.
5. Why is the immediate administration of oxygen under pressure (bag and mask) contraindicated for infants who are born with meconium-stained amniotic fluid?
6. Discuss the physiology of transient tachypnea.

■ Applying Your Knowledge

CASE STUDY

Mr. and Mrs. Boyd came to the hospital with Mrs. Boyd in active labor. She was 31 weeks pregnant and laboratory studies revealed an acute urinary tract infection. Fetal heart tones indicated fetal distress and Mrs. Boyd was prepared for a cesarean section. The Boyds had decided that the name of a male child would be Roy. Roy was born with an Apgar score of 4 and 6, weighing 1,980 g, and is preterm and small for gestational age. Six hours after birth, Roy's assessment reveals severe acrocyanosis, progressive metabolic disturbances, hematocrit of 56, and specific gravity of 1.005. The infant is in severe respiratory distress and his urinary output is 1 mL/kg/hr.

1. What types of circumstances are likely to contribute to Roy's respiratory distress (for example, related to method of delivery, maternal disease, newborn condition)?
2. What initial nursing actions would be implemented to address Roy's respiratory distress, and why?
3. Why might the physician order a plasma expander for Roy, and what nursing actions would be important when administering intravenous fluids to Roy?

4. Roy has to be intubated. Formulate a plan of care for the Boyd family identifying three nursing diagnoses to facilitate parent–infant bonding and listing the nursing order.

CRITICAL INQUIRY EXERCISE

1. Write a plan identifying the methods you would use to teach the mother how to implement a stimulation program at home for the preterm infant who has been deprived of environmental stimuli.

2. Identify all supporting devices and therapeutic procedures that might be used in direct support of an infant with respiratory distress syndrome. Synthesize how the devices and the procedures function to correct the pathologic processes demonstrated by assessment data and lab values.

CRITICAL EXPLORATION

1. Identify a preterm infant in the high-risk nursery. Examine the prenatal history and inpatient chart. Identify any existing factors that may have precipitated an early delivery.

2. Collaborate with two of your classmates to practice the sequential steps of external cardiac massage in the newborn using the cardiopulmonary resuscitation doll. Present your skill to the class and instructors with the assistance of your two partners.

■ Practicing for NCLEX

MULTIPLE-CHOICE QUESTIONS

Select the letter that corresponds to the best answer for each question.

1. Baby girl LaTrond is born with an Apgar score of 5 and 7. The infant is experiencing respiratory difficulty. The nurse's immediate goal for this infant would be to:
   A. Establish adequate circulatory pattern within 2 minutes
   B. Clear the airway and establish respirations in 2 minutes
   C. Prevent respiratory distress syndrome
   D. Obtain the oxygen concentration in the circulating blood volume

2. After therapeutic interventions, baby LaTrond is able to adequately expand her lungs. The amount of pressure that would enable her to continue to reinflate the alveoli of her lungs would be:
   A. 10 to 15 cm of water
   B. 15 to 20 cm of water
   C. 20 to 25 cm of water
   D. 25 to 20 cm of water

3. Which method would be most appropriate to stimulate initial respirations in the high-risk newborn?
   A. Spanking the buttocks
   B. Slapping the face
   C. Squeezing the thorax
   D. Rubbing the back

4. Baby Susan is about 21 hours old and has begun to exhibit signs and symptoms of respiratory compromise after an uneventful delivery and "normal" newborn assessment. The nurse's initial response would be to:
   A. Obtain blood gas levels and position the infant prone.
   B. Increase the flow of oxygen and position the infant in Trendelenburg position.
   C. Place the infant on her abdomen and lower the head of the bed.
   D. Raise the head of the crib 15 degrees and place the infant on her back.

5. An infant whose temperature is being maintained by a radiant heat source should have the probe or disk placed:
   A. Over a scapula area near the midscapular line
   B. On the abdomen between the umbilicus and the xiphoid process
   C. Over the rib cage between the costal structures
   D. Over the diaphragm below the lungs

6. Baby girl Lathasa, born vaginally, was determined to be large for gestational age. The nurse would assess this newborn carefully for:
   A. Increased intracranial pressure
   B. Hypothermia
   C. Decreased red blood levels (anemia)
   D. Hyperglycemia

7. An infant of a diabetic mother may demonstrate which of the following?
   A. Shrill, high-pitched cry
   B. Tremors, jitteriness, and irritability
   C. Fat, puffy, cushingoid face
   D. Overall wasting, sunken abdomen

8. On the third day in the nursery, Mr. and Mrs. Hubbard's newborn baby girl Rhonda is diagnosed with Rh incompatibility. The nurse understands that this is most likely the result of which of the following?
   A. The exchange of fetal and maternal blood in utero
   B. Rh-positive fetus and Rh-positive father
   C. Rh-negative mother and Rh-positive father
   D. Family history of a genetic disorder

9. Which of the following newborn characteristics would suggest that there was nutritional deprivation during fetal growth?
   A. Widely separated sutures
   B. Excessive lanugo
   C. Excessive brown fat
   D. Disproportionately small head to large body

10. When administering intravenous fluids to a high-risk newborn, the nurse should be cautious to avoid which of the following?
    A. Congestive heart failure
    B. Polycythemia
    C. Decreased intracranial hemorrhage
    D. Increased tissue perfusion

ALTERNATE FORMAT QUESTIONS

Fill in the Blank

Supply the missing term or the information requested.

1. Retinopathy of prematurity (ROP) is an acquired ocular disease that leads to ——— and is caused by vasoconstriction of immature retinal blood vessels.
2. Kernicterus occurs as a result of the deposit of ——————————————— in the brain.
3. The premature infant with anemia might benefit from the administration of ——— to protect the red blood cells from oxidation.
4. An infant who is exposed to continuous subnormal body temperatures has a potential to develop———.

Multiple-Answer Multiple Choice

Circle the letter(s) corresponding to the appropriate answer(s). Select all that apply.

1. Which of the following would the nurse need to incorporate in the plan of care for a newborn who is large for gestational age (LGA)?
   A. Anticipate that the LGA newborn will have strong sucking ability.
   B. Be alert for respiratory problems due to increased intracranial pressure placing pressure on the respiratory center.
   C. Decrease feedings with the newborn who is LGA to reduce size and prevent obesity.
   D. Observe LGA infants closely for signs of hyperbilirubinemia.
   E. Decrease stimulation such as holding and talking to the infant who is LGA to prevent seizures.
   F. Assess for possible impaired parenting due to newborn's high-risk status.

UNIT VI

The Nursing Role in Health Promotion for a Childrearing Family

CHAPTER 27

Principles of Growth and Development

CHAPTER OVERVIEW

Chapter 27 examines and summarizes the basic concepts of hereditary and environmental factors that influence a child's growth and development. The theories of development according to Freud, Erikson, Piaget, and Kohlberg are discussed. The chapter also explores the developmental tasks of parenting as the child progresses through various growth stages. The implications of growth and development for the nursing care of children from various age groups are explored, and interviewing and therapeutic communication skills needed by the nurse when caring for children in various stages of growth and development are also discussed. A case study presents a contrasting view of the developmental characteristics for each stage.

LEARNING OBJECTIVES

After mastering the content in this chapter, you should be able to do the following:

1. Describe principles of growth and development and developmental stages according to major theorists.
2. Assess a child to determine the stage of development the child has reached.
3. Formulate nursing diagnoses that address wellness as well as both a potential for delay and an actual delay in growth and development.
4. Identify expected outcomes for nursing goals for a growing child.
5. Plan nursing interventions to assist a child in achieving and maintaining normal growth and development.
6. Implement nursing actions such as providing age-appropriate play materials to support normal growth and development patterns.
7. Evaluate outcomes to be certain that nursing goals related to growth and development have been achieved.
8. Identify National Health Goals related to growth and development that nurses can be instrumental in helping the nation to achieve.
9. Identify areas of nursing care related to growth and development that could benefit from additional nursing research or application of evidence-based practice.
10. Use critical thinking to analyze factors that influence growth and development and ways to strengthen paths to achieving a new developmental stage.
11. Integrate knowledge of growth and development with the nursing process to achieve quality maternal and child health nursing care.

KEY TERMS

abstract thought
accommodation
adaptability
approach
assimilation
attention span
autonomy versus shame
centering
cognitive development
concrete operational thought
conservation
conventional development
development
developmental milestone
developmental task
distractibility
egocentrism
formal operational thought
growth
industry versus inferiority
identity versus role confusion
initiative versus guilt
integrity versus despair
intuitive thought
libido
macronutrient theory
maturation
micronutrient
mood quality
permanence
postconventional development
preoperational thought
prereligious stage
reversibility
rhythmicity
role fantasy
schema
sensorimotor stage
temperament
threshold of response
trust versus mistrust

■ Mastering the Information

MATCHING:

Match the terms in Column I with a definition, example, or related statement from Column II. Place the letter corresponding to the answer in the space provided.

COLUMN I

1. _____Genetic makeup
2. _____Temperament
3. _____Parent–child relationship
4. _____Latent phase
5. _____Socioeconomic level
6. _____Postconventional development

COLUMN II

A. A time in which a child's libido is diverted into concrete thinking
B. Possible interference in parents' ability to provide adequate health care and nutrition
C. A child's inherited background
D. A stage of cognitive development displayed by adolescents as they begin to have abstract thoughts about standards of conduct
E. An individual child's particular manner of thinking, behaving, or reacting to environmental stimuli
F. Loss of this crucial environmental influence can interfere with a child's growth and development.

COLUMN I PIAGET'S STAGES OF DEVELOPMENT

1. _____Sensorimotor
2. _____Preoperational thought
3. _____Intuitive thought
4. _____Concrete operational thought
5. _____Formal operational thought

COLUMN II

A. Thinking in terms of what could be rather than what currently exists
B. Inductive reasoning, from specific to general
C. Development of the concept of permanence and goal-directed behavior
D. Object viewed as having only one characteristic
E. Symbolic thought, egocentric and static thinking

SHORT ANSWER

Supply the missing term or the information requested.

1. ——— is a synonym for development.
2. ——— is a term used to express an increase in physical size or a quantitative change.
3. ——— denotes an increase in skill or the ability to function.
4. ——— is a term used to describe the child's intellectual abilities.
5. Complete the chart by naming the five psychoanalytic stages of development as defined by Sigmund Freud. Assign the appropriate childhood division and age range to these stages (see example).

Stage	Childhood	Division	Age Range
1.	Oral stage	Infant	1 month to 1 year
2.	______	______	______
3.	______	______	______
4.	______	______	______
5.	______	______	______

6. Identify the psychosocial stage of development identified by Erikson that is described by each of the following statements.

a. ——— Strives to obtain a sense of independence, taking pride in new accomplishments and wanting to do everything for himself/herself

b. ——— Expends effort to gain a sense of identity, bringing together experiences previously learned

c. ——— Concentrates on perfecting learned skills while seeking to enlarge his or her environment with school and community

d. ——— Recognizes that needs are met as they arise, with discomfort being quickly removed

e. ——— Learns how to do things, and the need for freedom and opportunity to initiate motor skills increases

Stages of Moral Development

State the appropriate stage of moral development described in the sentences below.

1. ——— Imitates behavior and practices doing gestures only for gestures in return
2. ——— Internalizes standards of conduct, doing what he or she thinks is right regardless of an existing social rule
3. ——— Learns that certain actions may elicit positive or negative behaviors from parents
4. ——— Punishment-obedience orientation, governed easily by parental authority
5. ——— Behaviors are influenced more by what is "nice" than by what may be right or wrong

■ Applying Your Knowledge

CASE STUDY:

Consider the most recent pediatric patient for whom you have provided nursing care in the clinical environment. Note the cognitive, psychosocial, and moral stages of the child's development.

1. Write a summary of the characteristics that you were able to identify for each of these stages. Include how the patient demonstrated each stage of development.

2. Indicate whether the stage of development was appropriate for the child's chronologic age.

3. Evaluate your assessment by writing a rationale as to why you think the patient did or did not meet the developmental task for each of the stages.

CRITICAL INQUIRY EXERCISE

1. Write a teaching plan that could be used to prepare the parents of a 13-month-old for the next stage of the child's development.
2. Compile a list of potentially dangerous areas in the average household environment that would be accessible to a toddler. Write to the nearest pediatric hospital's education department to obtain the information that they provide to their clients and families on safety and anticipatory guidance.

CRITICAL EXPLORATION

Choose a stage of childhood and interview a parent with a child in that age range. Attempt to identify the type of temperament reactivity pattern manifested by the child in each of the nine categories and evidence that the parent has, or has not, met the developmental tasks of parenting for the child's developmental stage.

■ Practicing for NCLEX

MULTIPLE-CHOICE QUESTIONS

Circle the letter that corresponds to the best answer for each question.

1. Mrs. Peters complains that her daughter Millie, age 1 month, is very fussy and will not sit in her car seat. She states that Millie never responds well to new people or toys. The nurse should explain which of the following to Mrs. Peters?
   A. When children are ill they are often fussy and respond poorly to new stimuli; these children often need to be hospitalized.
   B. Children have different approaches to life, and some children naturally demonstrate withdrawal when faced with new stimuli.
   C. The behavior she describes is a sign of Millie's rhythmicity and activity level, which are inborn reactivity patterns.
   D. Infants are seldom adaptable to new stimuli; as time passes Millie will probably have a less intense reaction to stimuli.

2. Jason is 2 months old. His mother reports that he wiggles and squirms constantly in his crib and wakes up at different times every day. The nurse recognizes these behaviors as examples of which of the following reaction patterns?
   A. Adaptability and attention span
   B. Distractibility and approach
   C. Mood and reaction intensity
   D. Activity and rhythmicity

3. When discussing temperament reactivity patterns of children with parents, which of the following would the nurse include?
   A. Early training and instruction can correct a child's apprehensive approach to new stimuli.
   B. Even children with poor adaptability can be expected to become accustomed to a new environment by the third exposure to the area.
   C. While some children will accept a substitute toy when crying for their favorite toy, others may refuse to accept anything else.
   D. Children who spend only 1 to 2 minutes with a toy before wanting a new one are usually mentally ill and sociopathic to a small degree.

4. When discussing care for Winston, who is 15 months old, with his mother, the nurse should consider the developmental tasks of parenting for which of the following divisions of childhood?
   A. Toddler
   B. Neonate
   C. Infant
   D. Preschooler

5. The nurse might discuss which of the following with the parents of Ida, a 2-year-old, during a parenting workshop?
   A. Ida can be expected to be cooperative and easily controlled at this stage of development.
   B. Ida may prefer finger foods and clothing she can put on without assistance at this age.
   C. Expect Ida to want to be held and cuddled a great deal at this stage of her development.
   D. At this age, Ida will take the initiative in activities and will question everything.

6. A key developmental task of parenting is learning to determine if a child is crying from hunger, discomfort, or some other reason. This task is most important for parents of a(n):
   A. Preschooler
   B. Infant
   C. Toddler
   D. School-age child

7. When planning the care of a 4-month-old child hospitalized with a respiratory tract infection and placed on strict bed rest, the nurse would include interventions to promote growth and development due to the child's:
   A. Decreased exposure to appropriate stimulation
   B. Reduced opportunities for initiative development
   C. Overexposure to varied stimuli
   D. Limited opportunities for independence

8. An appropriate goal when caring for a 4-year-old hospitalized child might be:
   A. The child will demonstrate initiative, within limits, evidenced by asking for paper and crayons to draw a picture.
   B. The parents will demonstrate appropriate parenting task achievement by dressing and feeding the child each day.
   C. The child will demonstrate formal operational thought by discussing the importance of being in the hospital.
   D. The parents will demonstrate the ability to interpret the child's behavioral cues.

ALTERNATE FORMAT QUESTIONS:

Fill in the Blank

Supply the missing term or the information requested.

1. ——— and ——— are essential physical data when making an assessment and should be accurately plotted on a growth chart.
2. ——— ———includes provision of information regarding further expectation of a child's ability to function in his/her environment.

Multiple-Answer Multiple Choice

Circle the letter(s) corresponding to the appropriate answer(s). Select all that apply.

1. The parents of an adolescent:
   A. Must set strict limits on activities to prevent the child from becoming independent and taking initiative
   B. Often experience difficulty in becoming independent of their child's life and in developing their own interests again
   C. Should not offer support or help to the child during this stage, so the child can develop a sense of independence
   D. Must take an active authoritarian role in planning the child's daily activities and future experiences
   E. Should educate their child about the long-term consequences of alcohol use

2. The nurse would determine that the parents of a preschooler had achieved their developmental tasks if which of the following behaviors were noted?
   A. The mother and father alternate attending kindergarten with the child each day.
   B. The child is allowed to play without limits in the home to encourage free expression and growth.
   C. The mother or father sits with the child and sips imaginary tea from a toy teacup.
   D. The child is punished for talking too much and asking too many questions.
   E. The child is not punished when masturbation is exhibited.

CHAPTER 28

The Family with an Infant

CHAPTER OVERVIEW

This chapter discusses the growth and development patterns of the infant and family. Emphasis is placed on specific growth and development parameters and common health deviations that should be assessed during routine child health visits. Nursing interventions aimed at family support, anticipatory guidance, and alleviating common health problems are highlighted. The case study explores appropriate interventions and rationales during a well-child visit in a health facility.

LEARNING OBJECTIVES

After mastering the content in this chapter, you should be able to do the following:

1. Describe normal infant growth and development and associated parental concerns.
2. Assess an infant for normal growth and development milestones.
3. Formulate nursing diagnoses related to infant growth and development and associated parental concerns.
4. Identify outcomes to promote optimal infant growth and development and health.
5. Plan nursing care to meet the infant's growth and development needs.
6. Implement nursing care related to normal growth and development of the infant.
7. Evaluate outcomes for achievement of optimal growth and development and effectiveness of care.
8. Identify National Health Goals related to infant growth and development that nurses can be instrumental in helping the nation achieve.
9. Identify areas related to nursing care of the infant that could benefit from additional nursing research or application of evidence-based practice.
10. Use critical thinking to analyze methods of care for the infant to be certain care is family-centered.
11. Integrate knowledge of infant growth and development with the nursing process to achieve quality maternal and child health nursing care.

KEY TERMS

baby-bottle syndrome
binocular vision
coordination of secondary schema
deciduous teeth
eighth-month anxiety
extrusion reflex
fine motor development
gross motor development
hand regard
Landau reflex
natal teeth
neck-righting reflex
neonatal teeth
object permanence
parachute reaction
pincer grasp
prehensile ability
primary circular reaction
seborrhea
secondary circular reaction
social smile
thumb opposition
ventral suspension

■ Mastering the Information

MATCHING

Match the description in Column I with the appropriate age from Column II. Place the letter corresponding to the answer in the space provided.

COLUMN I

1. _____Laughs out loud
2. _____Uses palmar grasp
3. _____Says first word, "da-da"
4. _____Pulls self to a standing position
5. _____Shows beginning stranger anxiety
6. _____Brings hands together and pulls at clothes
7. _____Sits securely without support
8. _____Can draw a semi-straight line with a crayon

COLUMN II

A. 3 months
B. 4 months
C. 6 months
D. 7 months
E. 8 months
F. 9 months
G. 10 months
H. 12 months

SHORT ANSWER

Supply the missing term or the information requested.

1. State four benefits derived from well-child follow-up visits.
2. What is the most serious complication for infants with supernumerary teeth?
3. Identify the four body positions from which to assess gross motor development in an infant.
4. List three ways parents can childproof their homes.
5. Identify two benefits to the growth and development of infants that may be promoted when bathing the infant.
6. How can parents provide tooth and oral care for their infants?
7. State three ways to prevent diaper dermatitis.
8. State three common causes of constipation.
9. What are three factors that should be assessed when an infant is experiencing diarrhea?

■ Applying Your Knowledge

CASE STUDY

Stephen is a 5-month-old infant visiting the well-child clinic for his second series of immunizations.

1. Stephen weighed 7 lb and was 20 inches long at birth. Based on normal growth and development parameters, what should his weight be at this visit?
2. List a normal set of vital signs that may be assessed from Stephen.
3. On what physiologic principle might the physician prescribe a vitamin with iron?
4. Stephen's mother is eager to feed him solid foods and asks the nurse if it would be recommended. What response would the nurse give? Why?

CRITICAL INQUIRY EXERCISE

1. Formulate a nursing care plan for the following case scenario: David, a 7-month-old infant, is experiencing diarrhea. His weight was 18 lb before the diarrhea; now it is 16 lb. His anterior fontanel is slightly sunken and mucous membranes are dry; urine output is diminished and the specific gravity is 1.035.
2. Contrast the developmental milestones occurring during infancy relating to fine and gross motor skills and physiologic and cognitive development.

CRITICAL EXPLORATION

Assess two infants of the same chronologic age, but one born at term and one born 2 to 3 months prematurely. Assess the developmental behaviors that are seen in the adjusted chronologic age groups for these infants. Compare the infants' performances. What principles of growth and development should be researched for this exercise?

■ Practicing for NCLEX

MULTIPLE-CHOICE QUESTIONS

Circle the letter that corresponds to the best answer for each question.

1. During a routine well-child visit the nurse should educate the parents regarding:
   A. The infant's need for meat by 4 months of age
   B. Expected growth and development patterns
   C. Specific yearly milestones the child must meet
   D. Signs and symptoms of failure to thrive

2. According to Erikson's theory of emotional development, infants will develop a sense of trust when:
   A. They can identify their mother and father
   B. They feel a sense of belonging, accepted as part of the family
   C. They can predict what is coming and their needs are consistently met
   D. Nutritional and hygiene needs are met on a daily basis

3. Keeping in mind the leading cause of accidents in infants, the nurse should advise parents to:
   A. Buy clothes for the infant with buttons rather than snaps
   B. Check all toys for small removable parts
   C. Provide round, cylinder-type toys
   D. Avoid finger foods before the age of 15 months

4. Since falls are a common cause of injury to infants, parents should be advised to:
   A. Avoid using pillows around the infant placed on a bed
   B. Use an infant seat when placing the infant on a table top
   C. Use blankets around the infant on a couch
   D. Place protective gates at the top and bottom of stairs

5. Palliative measures aimed at relieving colic should include:
   A. Placing a warm heating pad on the abdomen
   B. Diluting the formula
   C. Administering simethicone at 30-minute intervals
   D. Sitting the infant upright for a half-hour after feedings

6. Alice is 4 months of age. Her mother is singing to her. What type of response should be expected of Alice?
   A. Imitating the sounds
   B. Smiling, cooing, and gurgling
   C. Saying "da-da"
   D. Watching her mother's face without making a sound

7. At what age should an infant begin to locate an object hidden under a blanket?
   A. 6 months
   B. 8 months
   C. 10 months
   D. 12 months

8. When assessing the visual ability of a 7-month-old boy, the nurse should:
   A. Attempt to place a familiar object in the infant's hand and observe his response
   B. Use a brightly colored object and check the infant's ability to follow it
   C. Use a mirror to observe the infant's response to his image
   D. Observe the infant's ability to follow hand motions

9. When teaching parents about their infant's need for sleep, the nurse would be correct in stating that most infants usually sleep:
   A. 10 to 12 hours per night, with one or more naps
   B. 14 to 16 hours per night, with one nap
   C. An average of 18 to 20 hours each day
   D. At 4-hour intervals and throughout the night

10. What type of device would enhance the development of an 8-month-old infant through play activity?
    A. Stroller
    B. Floor mat
    C. Crib
    D. Play pen

11. A major developmental task for the family of an infant girl should be:
    A. Interpreting her cues to decipher her needs
    B. Allowing her to gain her autonomy and freedom to express herself
    C. Providing an environment for learning new skills
    D. Allowing her to take initiative and respond to her environment

12. An 8-month-old infant who loves to suck her thumb visits the clinic. Her mother is very worried that this habit will cause permanent dental problems. What should the nurse suggest to the mother?
    A. Wrap the infant's thumb with adhesive tape.
    B. Distract the infant with toys.
    C. Ignore this behavior.
    D. Remove the infant's thumb from her mouth as often as possible.

ALTERNATE FORMAT QUESTIONS

Fill in the Blank

Supply the missing term or the information requested.

1. At what age does an infant's immune system becomes functional? ____________________
2. The first tooth eruption is expected at what age?
   ____
3. Tracey, a 6-month-old, is undergoing a hearing assessment. Would you expect her to be able to locate sounds made at a distance over her head?
   ____

Multiple-Answer Multiple Choice

Circle the letter(s) corresponding to the appropriate answer(s). Select all that apply.

1. Parents report their infant daughter frequently wakes up from a sound sleep. What should the nurse advise the parents to do to help the child sleep through the night?
   A. When the infant awakens, wait a while and let her fall back to sleep.
   B. Go to the child immediately when she awakens and comfort her back to sleep.
   C. Provide soft music or toys to allow her to play quietly alone.
   D. Pick her up and rock her back to sleep.
   E. Place pillows around the infant to cushion the crib.
2. Patrick is 10 months old. What type of play activity is appropriate for his expected level of development?
   A. Rolling a ball
   B. Shaking a rattle
   C. Winding up a toy
   D. Playing patty-cake
   E. Peek-a-boo
   F. Playing with marbles

CHAPTER 29

The Family with a Toddler

CHAPTER OVERVIEW

This chapter explores the patterns of normal growth and development of the toddler. The developmental accomplishments related to fine and gross motor skills and language skills are presented. Anticipatory guidance with reference to making the toddler's environment safe is also addressed. The case study provides the student with the opportunity to provide teaching for the parents of a toddler through a teaching plan for health promotion.

LEARNING OBJECTIVES

After mastering the content in this chapter, you should be able to do the following:

1. Describe normal growth and development of the toddler period as well as common parental concerns.
2. Assess a toddler for normal growth and development milestones.
3. Formulate nursing diagnoses related to toddler growth and development or parental concerns regarding development.
4. Identify expected outcomes for nursing care of the toddler.
5. Plan nursing care to meet the toddler's growth and development needs, such as anticipatory guidance to prevent problems such as sleep disturbances, temper tantrums, or inappropriate toilet training practices.
6. Implement nursing care to promote normal growth and development of the toddler, such as discussing toddler developmental milestones with parents.
7. Evaluate goal outcomes established for care to be certain nursing goals associated with growth and development have been achieved.
8. Identify National Health Goals related to the toddler age group that nurses can be instrumental in helping the nation to achieve.
9. Identify areas related to care of the toddler that could benefit from additional nursing research or application of evidence-based practice.
10. Use critical thinking to analyze methods of care for the toddler to be certain care is family-centered.
11. Integrate knowledge of toddler growth and development with the nursing process to achieve quality maternal and child health nursing care.

KEY TERMS

assimilation
autonomy
deferred imitation
discipline
lordosis
parallel play
preoperational thought
punishment
tertiary circular reaction stage

■ Mastering the Information

MATCHING

Match the terms in Column I with a definition, example, or related statement from Column II. Place the letter corresponding to the answer in the space provided.

COLUMN I

1. ______Deferred imitation
2. ______Negativism
3. ______Separation anxiety
4. ______Lordosis
5. ______Discipline
6. ______Preoperational thought

COLUMN II

a. Universal fear that begins at about 6 months of age and persists throughout the preschool period

b. Remembering an action to mimic at a later time
c. A forward curve of the spine at the sacral area
d. A positive stage in toddler development; the toddler sees himself or herself as a separate individual with separate needs
e. Major period of cognitive development that usually occurs at the end of the toddler period
f. Setting rules to teach children what is expected of them

SHORT ANSWER

Supply the missing term or the information requested.

1. Describe the gross motor, language, and play developmental milestones that are accomplished at ages 15, 24, and 30 months.
2. Allowing self-feeding is a major way to strengthen ________________ in a toddler.

■ Applying Your Knowledge

CASE STUDY

Mr. and Mrs. Stargell and their 18-month-old son, Cody, are being seen today in the pediatrician's office where you are a nurse for a follow-up visit. The night before, Mr. Stargell discovered that Cody had tumbled down the stairs. The Stargells called the emergency room at a local children's hospital; they were instructed to bring Cody to the ER immediately. Cody was given a thorough examination and was treated for a small laceration to the head and a severely sprained arm. He was discharged in stable condition from the ER with instructions to see the pediatrician the following morning.

1. What information regarding toddler safety should you include in your plan to teach health promotion to Cody's parents?
2. You begin your assessment of Cody with a careful health history. What is the rationale for taking this health history?
3. Explain how information from a health history will help you develop a teaching plan for Cody's parents.

CRITICAL INQUIRY EXERCISE

1. Formulate a nursing care plan that will focus on setting safety guidelines for an 18-month-old child in the home environment.
2. List outcome criteria that might be established before the parents leave the pediatrician's office.

CRITICAL EXPLORATION

1. Visit a day-care setting and observe a group of toddlers during a free play period for 30 minutes or more. Select one toddler from the group and describe how he or she plays among the group members.
2. Visit the Red Cross center in your community and obtain the name and address of an agency that will furnish literature to institutions or families on poison prevention and child safety. Write for the literature and ask your instructor for assistance to distribute the materials to the parents of the children at your pediatric clinical site.

■ Practicing For NCLEX

MULTIPLE-CHOICE QUESTIONS

Circle the letter that corresponds to the best answer for each question.

1. The child's universal language is:
   A. Behavior
   B. Crying
   C. Touching
   D. Play

2. Which of the following describes the type of play observed with toddlers?
   A. Solitary
   B. Parallel
   C. Competitive
   D. Fantasy

3. When developing a plan of care to reduce the incidence of lead poisoning, which of the following would be most important for the nurse to include?
   A. Parent education
   B. Early detection
   C. Family planning
   D. Chelating therapy

4. Which of the following would the nurse be least likely to assess in a child with lead poisoning?
   A. Irritability
   B. Cardiomegaly
   C. Headaches
   D. Abominal pain

5. When planning the care for a toddler who is to be hospitalized, the nurse plans interventions based on minimizing the toddler's emotional stress related to which of the following?
   A. Loss of control
   B. Fear of bodily injury
   C. Fear of death
   D. Separation anxiety

6. Which of the following would the nurse suggest as appropriate for promoting adequate toddler nutrition?
   A. Use of skim milk after age 2
   B. Unrestricted fat intake until age 3
   C. Daily calorie intake of 1,300 kcal
   D. Limited exposure to finger foods

ALTERNATE FORMAT QUESTIONS

Fill in the Blank

Supply the missing term or the information requested.

1. The toddler has the developmental task of achieving greater ____________ and less dependence.

2. ________ is the type of accident that occurs most frequently in toddlers.

Multiple-Answer Multiple Choice

Circle the letter(s) corresponding to the appropriate answer(s). Select all that apply.

1. Which interventions would be most appropriate for a toddler?
   A. Leaving toddlers alone in the tub for a brief moment while bathing them
   B. Offering high-protein snacks rather than high-carbohydrate snacks
   C. Placing a gate on the door to a toddler's room
   D. Informing parents that sleep times will be shorter for toddlers than for infants
   E. Offering a toddler something pleasurable in the middle of a temper tantrum to stop the tantrum
   F. Assisting the child in putting his clothes on correctly to develop neatness
   G. Placing medicines on shelves at least 4 feet high so they are out of a child's reach
   H. Encouraging parents to buy arch-supportive shoes
   I. Beginning attempts at potty-training around the age of 2 years or so
   J. Choosing a potty-chair that sits on the commode

CHAPTER 30

The Family with a Preschooler

CHAPTER OVERVIEW

Preschool-age children demonstrate the desire to care for themselves through daily activities. They insist on dressing themselves and often resist assistance from parents. The nurse should include the need for parent education related to these behaviors when planning nursing care. This chapter discusses the developmental tasks and anticipatory guidance for children in this age group. The case study provides a learning opportunity for sex education during the preschool years.

LEARNING OBJECTIVES

After mastering the content in this chapter, you should be able to do the following:

1. Describe normal growth and development as well as common parental concerns of the preschool period.
2. Assess a preschooler for normal growth and developmental milestones.
3. Formulate nursing diagnoses related to preschool growth and development and common parental concerns.
4. Identify expected outcomes for nursing care of the toddler.
5. Plan nursing care to meet the preschooler's growth and development needs, such as planning age-appropriate play activities.
6. Implement nursing care related to normal growth and development of the preschooler, such as preparing a preschooler for an invasive procedure.
7. Evaluate outcome criteria established for care to be certain normal growth and development goals have been achieved.
8. Identify National Health Goals related to the preschool period that nurses can be instrumental in helping the nation to achieve.
9. Identify areas related to care of the preschool-age child that could benefit from additional nursing research or application of evidence-based practice.
10. Use critical thinking to analyze additional ways in which growth and developmental problems of the preschool child can be prevented and care can be family-centered.
11. Integrate knowledge of preschool growth and development with the nursing process to achieve quality maternal and child health nursing care.

KEY TERMS

broken fluency	endomorphic body build
bruxism	genu valgus
conservation	intuitional thought
ectomorphic body build	Oedipus complex
Electra complex	secondary stuttering

■ Mastering the Information

MATCHING

Match the terms in Column I with a definition, example, or related statement from Column II. Place the letter corresponding to the answer in the space provided.

COLUMN I

1. _____Initiative
2. _____Play
3. _____Regression
4. _____Broken fluency
5. _____Intuitional thought

COLUMN II

a. Reverting to behaviors practiced in earlier years
b. Repetition and prolongation of sounds
c. Method by which preschoolers use their imagination

d. Lacking insight to view themselves as others see them and thinking of themselves as always right
e. Achievement leading to knowledge that learning new things is fun

SHORT ANSWER

Supply the missing term or the information requested.

1. Define the following terms: endomorphic; ectomorphic; genu valgus; bruxism.
2. Describe the Oedipus and Electra complexes.
3. Explain how the preschooler's inability to understand the law of conservation may affect your ability to care for him or her.
4. What are some therapeutic methods that can be practiced by the nurse and family to alleviate the preschooler's fear of the dark?
5. Identify four basic rules recommended to resolve secondary stuttering.

■ Applying Your Knowledge

CASE STUDY

Mrs. Bell and her two children, Amy (age 8) and Bryan (age 4), are visiting the health center today for a well-child appointment. Mrs. Bell is 6 months pregnant. After the physician's visit, Mrs. Bell asks if she could speak with you for a few moments about Bryan. She explains that she is very concerned about Bryan's fixation on his genitals. Mrs. Bell began to notice this behavior about 2 weeks after she enrolled him in a day-care center. She says that he masturbates often and seems to have forgotten what the family has taught him about his "private parts."

1. What is the developmental theory that would suggest why Bryan has started to demonstrate this behavior?
2. What guidelines would you use to advise Mrs. Bell regarding Bryan's masturbating in public?
3. What basic rule concerning sex education should you be sure to mention to help protect Bryan from sexual abuse?
4. Outline a teaching plan to help the mother explain pregnancy and the arrival of a new baby.

CRITICAL INQUIRY EXERCISE

1. Contrast the developmental milestones across the life span of the 3-, 4-, and 5-year-old.
2. Prepare a teaching plan for the parent and preschooler about developing safety measures in the home.

CRITICAL EXPLORATION

1. Visit a kindergarten and talk with a preschool child near the end of the day. Ask the child to tell you what happened during the day. Assess the child's language development, understand how the term "egocentrism" applies to the preschooler, and identify if the child is accomplishing the developmental tasks of that age group.
2. Visit a preschool child who is hospitalized for an elective surgery. Talk to the child before the surgery. Obtain three or four pictures depicting a pediatric hospital area, including the patient's room and the operating room. Do not include any pictures suggestive of invasive procedures or treatment. Show these pictures to the preschooler and ask him or her to make up a story about the pictures. Record the story as the preschooler talks to you. Identify the statements indicating fear and stress. Notice in the story how the child's ability to fantasize allows him or her to stretch the imagination to include even mutilation, although the pictures do not suggest aggressive or invasive subjects.

■ Practicing for NCLEX

MULTIPLE-CHOICE QUESTIONS

Circle the letter that corresponds to the best answer for each question.

1. Which of the following types of play is primarily demonstrated by preschoolers?
   A. Parallel
   B. Imaginary
   C. Solitary
   D. Cooperative

2. When preparing a preschooler for an invasive procedure, the nurse would plan interventions to address which fear?
   A. Fear of the dark
   B. Fear of abandonment
   C. Fear of losing control
   D. Fear of mutilation

3. Which action would be most appropriate to help lessen the feelings of rivalry among siblings?
   A. Punish for unacceptable behavior.
   B. Separate siblings and give individual attention separately.
   C. Interact with younger and older siblings together.
   D. Allow the older sibling to practice adult roles to comfort him or her.

4. A preschooler appropriately explores his body by:
   A. Dressing up in parents' clothing
   B. Masturbating
   C. Inflicting harm
   D. Comparing his body parts with playmates

5. Which of the following is an appropriate activity for the preschooler?
   A. Cutting paper dolls
   B. Playing house
   C. Stacking blocks
   D. Dart board game

ALTERNATE FORMAT QUESTIONS

Fill in the Blank

Supply the missing term or the information requested.

1. The developmental task for the preschool-age child is to achieve a sense of ____________________

2. ________ ________ refers to the strong emotional attachment of a preschool boy to his mother.

Multiple-Answer Multiple Choice

Circle the letter(s) corresponding to the appropriate answer(s). Select all that apply.

1. Which of the following are appropriate nursing interventions for a preschooler?
   A. Encourage the preschooler to speak during the health examination.
   B. Assess weight and height on a standard growth chart at each health visit.
   C. Include head circumference on each physical examination.
   D. Encourage constructive play.
   E. Provide a helmet for bicycle riding.
   F. Avoid parental use of medications while child is watching.
   G. Turn the water heater to 110° to 120°F.
   H. Allow the preschooler to floss his or her teeth at least once a day.
   I. Keep a dim light on in the child's room at night.
   J. Provide the preschooler with a private space for his or her belongings that is not to be shared.:

CHAPTER 31

The Family with a School-Age Child

CHAPTER OVERVIEW

The school-age years (ages 6 to 12) represent a time of slow physical growth, but cognitive and developmental growth is rapid. When caring for this age group, it is important to stress the physical growth and accomplishment of emotional, cognitive, and moral developmental tasks. The school-age period is the time the child becomes independent and begins to separate from the family for long periods of time. The nurse should know the principles of development related to this age group to promote developmental needs and safety. This chapter contains exercises that help the student in learning developmental tasks and in assisting the family of a school-age child by providing anticipatory guidance. The case study emphasizes the principles of school-age growth and development.

LEARNING OBJECTIVES

After mastering the content in this chapter, you should be able to do the following:

1. Describe the normal growth and development pattern and common parental concerns of the school-age period.
2. Assess a school-age child for normal growth and development milestones.
3. Formulate nursing diagnoses for the family of a school-age child.
4. Identify expected outcomes based on health assessment findings.
5. Plan anticipatory guidance to prevent problems of growth and development in the school-age child (e.g., teaching about normal puberty).
6. Implement nursing care to help achieve normal growth and development of the school-age child, such as counseling parents about helping their child adjust to a new school.
7. Evaluate outcome criteria to be certain that goals of care have been achieved.
8. Identify National Health Goals related to the school-age child that nurses can be instrumental in helping the nation achieve.
9. Identify areas related to care of school-age children that could benefit from additional nursing research or application of evidence-based practice.
10. Use critical thinking to analyze ways in which the care of the school-age child can be more family-centered.
11. Integrate knowledge of school-age growth and development with the nursing process to achieve quality maternal and child health nursing care.

KEY TERMS

accommodation
caries
class inclusion
conservation
decenter
inclusion
latchkey child
malocclusion
nocturnal emissions
preconventional reasoning

■ Mastering the Information

MATCHING

Match the terms in Column I with a definition, example, or related statement from Column II. Place the letter corresponding to the answer in the space provided.

COLUMN I: CHRONOLOGIC SCHOOL AGE

1. _____Age 6
2. _____Age 7
3. _____Age 8
4. _____Age 9
5. _____Age 10
6. _____Age 11
7. _____Age 12

 Study Guide to Accompany Maternal and Child Health Nursing: Care of the Childbearing and Childrearing Family, revised reprint, fifth edition by Joyce Young Johnson and Edna Boyd-Davis.

COLUMN II: PHYSICAL OR PSYCHOSOCIAL DEVELOPMENT

a. Best friends important; whispering and giggling
b. Teacher as the authority figure
c. Social and cooperative
d. Conservation learned
e. Ready for competitive games
f. Clubs are formed, all boys or all girls
g. Insecure with members of opposite sex

SHORT ANSWER

Supply the missing term or the information.

1. For the first 1 to 2 years after menarche, most girls experience menstrual irregularity primarily because their cycle is ———. Cycles become more regular with the onset of ————————.
2. As seminal fluid is produced, boys begin to notice ejaculation during sleep, called ——— ———.
3. Compare and contrast the accomplishment or failure of the developmental task industry versus inferiority.
4. Describe the characteristics of the following forms of cognitive development: decenter; accommodation; conservation; class inclusion.
5. What advice would you give parents to improve or increase their child's interest in reading?
6. Define school phobia. Discuss why this occurs and give ways to help the family cope with and resolve these fears.
7. Describe measures that can be taken to avoid the following accidents with the school-age child: drowning; motor vehicle accidents; sports injuries; firearms.

■ Applying Your Knowledge

CASE STUDY

Mrs. Elway brings her daughter Clois, age 11, to the well-child care center for an annual check-up. The nurse obtains the history and begins the assessment. Clois's vital signs are within normal limits: temperature 98.6°F, pulse 75, respirations 26, blood pressure 110/58. Mrs. Elway tells the nurse she is concerned about Clois's sudden outbreaks of perspiration; although the episodes are not frequent, they don't seem to correlate with environmental temperatures.

1. What anticipatory guidance should the nurse give to Mrs. Elway regarding breast development and vaginal secretion?
2. Clois wants to play soccer at school; Mrs. Elway asks the nurse if she thinks this would be a good idea. What principles regarding structured activities should the nurse call upon to formulate a response?

CRITICAL INQUIRY EXERCISE

1. Develop a teaching plan for parents to explain the physical growth related to sexuality occurring during the school-age years.
2. Create a set of key points to discuss when providing anticipatory guidance for parents on detection of recreational drug use.

CRITICAL EXPLORATION

1. Observe students in an elementary school classroom. Record the behaviors of the teacher that may be considered positive and valuable to the children's transition to the school environment.
2. Observe several students for gross and fine motor development. Compare the findings to the expected motor development for that chronologic age group.
3. Visit a school during a recess period and observe the behaviors of children that are active with the following types of play: (a) group, (b) cooperative, (c) grouping, (d) same gender, and (e) consisting of rules.

■ Practicing for NCLEX

MULTIPLE-CHOICE QUESTIONS

Circle the letter that corresponds to the best answer for each question.

1. Sex education should be introduced at:
   A. High school
   B. Junior high school
   C. Middle school
   D. Grade/elementary school

2. Peer relationships are important to the school-age child. Which of the following is a characteristic of the 9-year-old?
   A. Boys and girls love to play together.
   B. Activities are very complete.
   C. Boys and girls begin to have social interactions.
   D. Loyalty and affiliation are directed to a same-sex peer groups.

3. Which of the following permanent teeth would the nurse expect to be present when assessing a 7-year old?
   A. Lower cuspids
   B. Upper central incisor
   C. First bicuspid
   D. Second molar

4. Which of the following is correct regarding physical maturation before puberty?
   A. Boys are usually taller than girls.
   B. Girls are usually taller than boys.
   C. Boys and girls are usually the same height.
   D. There is no pattern of height based on gender.

ALTERNATE FORMAT QUESTIONS

Fill in the Blank

Supply the missing term or the information requested.

1. Talent for music or art becomes evident and children respond well by age ___________.

Multiple-Answer Multiple Choice

Circle the letter(s) corresponding to the appropriate answer(s). Select all that apply.

1. Gross motor development will allow a 6-year-old to:
   A. Jump
   B. Tumble
   C. Skip rope well
   D. Play hopscotch
   E. Ride a bicycle

CHAPTER 32

The Family with an Adolescent

CHAPTER OVERVIEW

Chapter 32 provides an overview of adolescent growth and development, nursing care related to health promotion, and the management of illness in the adolescent. The physiologic and psychological needs of the adolescent and common health concerns encountered during adolescence are reviewed. The use of the nursing process to plan and provide appropriate health care for the adolescent and his or her family is explored.

LEARNING OBJECTIVES

After mastering the content in this chapter, you should be able to do the following:

1. Describe the normal growth and development patterns and common parental concerns of the adolescent period.
2. Assess adolescents for normal growth and development milestones.
3. Formulate nursing diagnoses for the family of an adolescent.
4. Identify expected outcomes based on health assessment findings.
5. Plan nursing care related to growth and development concerns of the adolescent, such as planning health teaching necessary to accept pubertal changes.
6. Implement nursing care related to growth and development or special needs of the adolescent, such as organizing a discussion group on ways to prevent drug abuse.
7. Evaluate expected outcomes to be certain that nursing care was comprehensive.
8. Identify National Health Goals related to the adolescent that nurses could be instrumental in helping the nation to achieve.
9. Identify areas related to care of adolescents that could benefit from additional nursing research or application of evidence-based practice.
10. Use critical thinking to analyze ways in which care of the adolescent could be more family-centered.
11. Integrate knowledge of adolescent growth and development with the nursing process to achieve quality maternal and child health nursing care.

KEY TERMS

adolescence
comedones
formal operations
glycogen loading
identity
puberty
role confusion
stalking
substance abuse

■ Mastering the Information

MATCHING

Match the terms in Column I with a definition, example, or related statement from Column II. Place the letter corresponding to the answer in the space provided.

COLUMN I

1. ____Adolescence
2. ____Formal operational thought
3. ____Empathy
4. ____Intimacy
5. ____Substance abuse
6. ____Puberty
7. ____Pustular acne
8. ____Runaway
9. ____Suicide
10. ____Secondary sex characteristics

COLUMN II

a. The physiologic period between the beginning of puberty and the cessation of bodily growth
b. Use of chemicals to improve the mental state

c. Deliberate self-injury with the intent to end one's life
d. Body hair configuration and breast growth distinguishing males from females
e. Feeling for another by projecting one's self into the other person's situation
f. Development of a sense of compassion or concern for others
g. The stage at which the individual first becomes capable of sexual reproduction
h. A 10- to 17-year-old absent from home at least overnight without permission of parent or guardian
i. Condition often treated with systemic antibiotics
j. Ability to think in abstract terms and use the scientific method

SHORT ANSWER

Supply the missing term or information requested.

1. One major dilemma encountered by adolescents that leads to many growth and development concerns is that they are ______ in some respects but still ______________ in others.
2. Early adolescence generally occurs between the ages of ________ and ________ years; middle adolescence occurs between ______ and ______ years; and late adolescence occurs between __________ and __________ years.
3. Cognitive development over the adolescent years involves the stage of ________ ________, which begins at age ________ or ________.
4. The goal of therapy for acne treatment is to decrease ________ ________, prevent ________, and control ________ ________.
5. As many as 90% of high school seniors report having used ______________.
6. Discuss two reasons the nurse should obtain an adolescent's health history in private, separately from his or her parents.
7. List three common factors (primary assessment areas) that explain why adolescents may suffer fatigue.
8. What major task must the adolescent achieve in each of the following developmental areas: sense of intimacy, emancipation from parents, and value system?
9. State two ways nurses can be instrumental in helping to achieve National Health Goals related to adolescent health.
10. Describe the common social behaviors manifested by adolescents at ages 13, 14, 15, 16, and 17.
11. Identify 7 of the 14 danger signs for adolescent suicide.

■ Applying Your Knowledge

CASE STUDY

Angelique Rodriguez, age 14, was referred to you, the school nurse, by her guidance counselor. Angelique's grades have dropped from A's to low C's over the past two semesters, and she has become aggressive and refuses to talk to the teachers or counselors. The counselor suspects drugs, pregnancy, or depression but doesn't know how to help Angelique.

1. What would three of your first actions be when approaching Angelique?
2. What permissions would you need from Angelique and her parents, and what actions could you take without contacting her parents?
3. If Angelique admitted depression and drug abuse, what initial steps would you take to get help for her?

CRITICAL INQUIRY EXERCISE

1. Prepare a teaching plan for an adolescent group that addresses methods for maintaining adequate nutrition, rest, and exercise.
2. How could the usual social behaviors noted in adolescents ages 13 through 17 contribute to problems or concerns that may be experienced by the adolescent and his or her family?

CRITICAL EXPLORATION

Attend a group session at an adolescent drug rehabilitation center. Note common themes related to why adolescents use drugs.

■ Practicing for NCLEX

MULTIPLE-CHOICE QUESTIONS

Circle the letter that corresponds to the best answer for each question.

1. Because of changes occurring in the sebaceous glands and sweat glands of adolescents, the nurse would include which of the following in health care teaching?
   A. Increased hygiene requirements to reduce body odor and acne
   B. Information regarding the need for increased fat-soluble vitamins
   C. Instructions regarding medications for inadequate sweat production
   D. Exercises that will minimize the production of sweat

2. When planning a teaching strategy for an adolescent, the nurse should do which of the following?
   A. Give information about how the teen can manage the specific problems he or she identifies.
   B. Maintain an air of authority by providing explanations for care procedures to parents only.
   C. Provide information related to long-term health needs, since adolescents respond best to long-range planning.
   D. Teach the parents first, since they will be better able to teach the teen.

3. At his physical, Bob, 14 years old, tells the nurse he is "a short, clumsy klutz." The nurse should respond in which of the following ways?
   A. Discuss with Bob the fact that his clumsiness is probably a sign of an easily curable disease.
   B. Instruct Bob in methods of relieving clumsiness through muscle exercises and improving nutrition.
   C. Explain to Bob that adolescent boys are usually taller than adolescent girls, so he should be examined.
   D. Inform Bob that what he is experiencing will lessen and he will become more coordinated as he grows taller over the next 4 to 6 years.

4. The mother of Sheila, age 13, reports that Sheila "talks for hours to her girlfriends, and spends most of her waking hours with girls." The nurse could reassure Sheila's mother by explaining which of the following?
   A. If Sheila spends less time on the phone during the next 2 years, she will mature normally.
   B. Sheila is probably talking to boys when her parents aren't around.
   C. Talking on the phone and spending time with girlfriends is normal for a girl of Sheila's age.
   D. There is no current threat of homosexuality due to Sheila's young age.

5. Marla is 15 years old. Marla's mother tells the nurse she fears that her daughter will get into serious trouble soon because she is always "going for a walk or sitting outside somewhere." The nurse should respond in which of the following ways to this information?
   A. Encourage Marla's mother to follow her to determine why Marla is being so distant.
   B. Inform the mother that Marla is probably all right and is seeking the privacy she needs.
   C. Schedule Marla for a blood and urine drug screening immediately.
   D. Tell Marla's mother to call a psychologist to help her deal with the stress of adolescence.

6. Which of the following would be a positive sign of identity formation in a client in late adolescence?
   A. Obtaining a job to save money
   B. Continuous dieting
   C. Getting pregnant and having a baby
   D. Living with parents

7. Daryl, age 17, states he shouldn't have sex and get girls pregnant "mostly because my parents would be really mad." Daryl's response may indicate a lack of development in which of the following areas?
   A. Cognitive development
   B. Moral development
   C. Physiologic development
   D. Religious development

8. Which of the following would be a realistic outcome criterion related to an adolescent with a history of experimentation with marijuana? The adolescent will:
   A. Stop using drugs immediately without assistance.
   B. Discuss ways to enjoy life without drugs.
   C. Use only marijuana, with no additional drug use.
   D. Smoke marijuana in moderation.

9. Which of the following would be a realistic outcome criterion related to an adolescent with a medical condition requiring a special diet?
   A. The adolescent with diabetes will eat no sweet, sugary foods.
   B. The adolescent with hypertension will not eat potato chips.
   C. The adolescent with fatigue will choose preferred foods high in vitamins and minerals.
   D. The adolescent with acne will discuss the need for foods high in lipids to replace the deficient body supply.

10. Anna, age 17, has been identified as a suicide risk. The nurse should watch her carefully and during discharge teaching discuss the need for the family to watch her particularly closely:
   A. Before the beginning of the school year
   B. Between noon and 3 p.m.
   C. During her menstrual period
   D. Late at night

ALTERNATE FORMAT QUESTIONS

Fill in the Blank

Supply the missing term or the information requested.

1. Females generally stop growing within ________ years from menarche.

2. Adolescents will experience a slight __________ in pulse rate as they move toward adulthood.

3. Adolescents will experience a slight __________ in blood pressure as they move toward adulthood.

Multiple-Answer Multiple Choice

Circle the letter(s) corresponding to the appropriate answer(s). Select all that apply.

1. Circle the appropriate nursing interventions for an adolescent who is abusing the specific drug.
   A. Alcohol: Investigate the presence of alcohol abuse by parents or other close family members.
   B. Amphetamines: Monitor for symptoms such as aggressive and demanding behavior and paranoia.
   C. Anabolic steroids: Instruct athletes that these drugs cause fatigue and depression, which will lead to weight gain.
   D. Barbiturates: Allow the suicide-prone adolescent the control of managing oral administration alone, since these are generally harmless drugs.
   E. Cigarettes: Have a nurse who smokes discuss with the teen the evils and problems caused by smoking as one who knows the problems personally.
   F. Cocaine/crack: Educate adolescents on the potential for immediate death even with the first use.
   G. LSD/PCP: Inform teens that this drug can cause brain damage and dangerous flashbacks.
   H. Marijuana: Emphasize that short-term use can cause pulmonary problems, although low but consistent use over several years has shown no harmful effects.
   I. Opiates: Discuss the potential for exposure to the AIDS virus when shared needles are used.
   J. All drugs: Emphasize the fact that there are no "good" drugs and all chemicals are harmful to the body to some extent.

CHAPTER 33

Child Health Assessment

CHAPTER OVERVIEW

This chapter offers an in-depth discussion of the nursing techniques used in child health assessment. Interviewing skills and procedures for performing physical and developmental assessments are described. Nursing interventions aimed at reducing the child's anxiety during assessment procedures are given. Normal growth and development parameters and health deviations are explained for each component of the health assessment. A case study is presented to help the student study the principles used in conducting an abdominal assessment.

LEARNING OBJECTIVES

After mastering the content in this chapter, you should be able to do the following:

1. State the purposes for health assessment in children of all ages.
2. Assess a child and family by health interview, physical examination, and development screening.
3. Use the nursing process to determine and address nursing diagnoses based on health assessment findings.
4. Identify National Health Goals related to health assessment of children that nurses can be instrumental in helping the nation achieve.
5. Identify areas related to health assessment of children that could benefit from additional nursing research.
6. Use critical thinking to analyze ways that health assessment skills can be incorporated into nursing care procedures.
7. Synthesize the nursing process with knowledge of health assessment to achieve quality maternal and child health nursing care.

KEY TERMS

audiogram
auscultation
bruit
chief concern
cognitive learning
conjunctivitis
deep tendon reflexes
diaphragmatic excursion
epispadias
esotropia
exotropia
fasciculations

general appearance
geographic tongue
gingivae
hordeolum
hydrocele
hypospadias

inspection
intelligence
intercostal spaces
kwashiorkor
palpation
percussion

physiologic splitting
point of maximum impulse
ptosis
retractions
review of systems
sinus arrhythmia
strabismus
superficial reflexes
temperament
tinea capitis
turgor
varicocele

■ Mastering the Information

MATCHING

Match the terms in Column I with a definition, example, or related statement from Column II. Place the letter corresponding to the answer in the space provided.

COLUMN I: BODY MASS INDEX INTERPRETATION

1. _____Underweight
2. _____Normal
3. _____Overweight
4. _____Obese

COLUMN II: BODY MASS INDEX FINDING

A. 32

B. 27

C. 20

D. 17.5

COLUMN I: CHILD HEALTH PROBLEMS

1. _____Iron deficiency anemia
2. _____Cyanosis
3. _____Endocarditis
4. _____Chromosomal abnormalities

COLUMN II: SIGNS AND SYMPTOMS THAT MAY BE NOTED ON THE EXTREMITIES

A. Simian crease

B. Concave nails

C. Clubbed fingers

D. Linear hemorrhages under the nails

SHORT ANSWER

Supply the missing term or the information requested.

1. Sinus arrhythmias are considered a normal phenomenon in children of __________ age. They are characterized by a marked heart rate increase on __________ and a marked heart rate decrease on ______________________________.
2. List and explain the nine categories for data gathering in performing the initial health assessment for the child and family.
3. What are the height and weight deviations that indicate failure to thrive syndrome in an infant?
4. Name two tests used to detect strabismus.
5. Describe the assessment technique used to detect choanal atresia.
6. Name three prominent features of chronic serous otitis media.

■ Applying Your Knowledge

CASE STUDY

Jennifer, age 14, is visiting the primary care center for a routine "return to school" physical. She will be examined by the physician to determine her diagnosis and any immediate care necessary.

1. What is an important consideration related to the examination and privacy that the nurse should be aware of regarding Jennifer?
2. On examination, how would the nurse divide the abdomen for inspection?
3. What would be the appearance of the abdomen if the contour and structure are normal?
4. Describe the sounds to be heard on auscultation.

CRITICAL INQUIRY EXERCISE

1. Pair off with another nursing student and practice performing an initial assessment using the eight categories for data gathering.
2. There is a significant change in the growth and development of the child moving from a toddler to a preschooler stage of development. Contrast the physical differences that you may find between the two groups of children.

CRITICAL EXPLORATION

1. Visit a well-child clinic or pediatrician's office and observe the performance of health assessments on children in various age groups. Focus on communication styles and techniques used by the parent, child, and health care provider.
2. Select a parent group, and explain to them why the Denver Developmental Screening Tool is used and how it is scored and interpreted.

■ Practicing for NCLEX

MULTIPLE-CHOICE QUESTIONS

Circle the letter that corresponds to the best answer for each question.

1. When obtaining information regarding the day history of a child, the nurse should ask:
   A. "How much food does your child normally eat?"
   B. "Does your child socialize well with others?"
   C. "Describe your child's normal sleep patterns."
   D. "What types of stools does your child normally have?"

2. Which of the following is a priority when performing a physical assessment on a newborn?
   A. Prevent squirming
   B. Maintain body temperature
   C. Examine the ears and throat before the eyes and nose
   D. Assess brachial pulse

3. When performing an assessment of the throat, depressing the tongue of a child who has acute epiglottititis is contraindicated because this:
   A. May precipitate upper airway obstruction
   B. Overstimulates the cough and gag reflex
   C. May be a source of bacterial infections
   D. May rupture the epiglottis

4. The most effective way to assess a toddler's gait is to:
   A. Observe play activity
   B. Perform a specific motor test
   C. Ask the child to walk with the parent
   D. Ask the child to hop on one foot

5. To assess hearing in a 1-month-old infant, the nurse should:
   A. Play a musical toy 4 feet from the infant's ear and observe for eye movement
   B. Repeat the infant's name in a soft tone and observe facial expressions
   C. Perform the Rinne test and observe for head turning
   D. Make a loud noise and observe for the startle reflex

6. When assessing a child's abdomen, which technique would the nurse perform first?
   A. Percussion
   B. Palpation
   C. Inspection
   D. Auscultation

7. An indication of bowel obstruction in the toddler is:
   A. Increased peristalsis with absence of stools for 2 or more days
   B. Abdominal distention with absence of peristalsis
   C. Severe abdominal pain with a loud bruit on auscultation
   D. Presence of an abdominal hernia with dry, foul-smelling stools

8. What would be an appropriate nursing assessment for a child who complains of a sore throat and dizziness?
   A. Otoscopic and throat exam
   B. Otoscopic and ophthalmic exam
   C. Mental status evaluation and complete neurologic exam
   D. Respiratory and cardiovascular system assessments

9. When performing an assessment for the presence of an inguinal hernia, which of the following should be considered a positive test result?
   A. Palpable femoral lymph nodes
   B. Extreme pain and discomfort in rectal and perineal area
   C. Bulging of the intestine while coughing
   D. Pelvic pain on palpation

10. To assess the school-age child for scoliosis the nurse should:
   A. Ask the child to stand straight with feet together
   B. Measure the leg lengths and pelvic girth
   C. Have the child bend over, inspecting for a dimpling
   D. Ask the child to walk to observe posture

11. Tina is a preschooler who is brought to the clinic by her mother for a check-up. Which of the following statements made by Tina's mother would most likely indicate that Tina has a vision problem?
    A. "Tina is always rubbing her eyes, blinking and squinting."
    B. "Tina sits so close to the television when she's watching it."
    C. "Tina still doesn't know her colors."
    D. "Tina doesn't seem to pay attention to what's in front of her."

12. To conduct the Denver Articulation Screening Examination (DASE), the nurse would ask the child to:
    A. Repeat some familiar words or phrases
    B. Read a favorite short story
    C. Recite a poem with age-appropriate words
    D. Read a phrase and interpret it

ALTERNATE FORMAT QUESTIONS

Fill in the Blank

1. The mobility of the eardrum (tympanic membrane) can be tested by injecting ________ into the ear canal.

2. ________ ________ is a rough-appearing tongue surface that accompanies general symptoms of illness such as fever.

Multiple-Answer Multiple Choice

Circle the letter(s) corresponding to the appropriate answer(s). Select all that apply.

1. Which of the following are high-risk conditions associated with hearing impairment in children?
    A. Perinatal infections
    B. High birthweight
    C. Hyperbilirubinemia
    D. Bacterial meningitis
    E. Anatomical malformation

2. Which statement(s) is correct regarding the assessment findings of the female genitalia?
    A. Hair growth in the pubic area typically appears triangular in shape.
    B. A vaginal discharge in a young child may be a sign of sexual abuse.
    C. An enlarged clitoris in an adolescent girl is a sign of sexual activity.
    D. Vaginal warts are common findings in most children under the age of 13.
    E. Pelvic examination is usually performed when the girl reaches 16 years of age.

CHAPTER 34

Communication and Teaching With Children and Families

CHAPTER OVERVIEW

Chapter 34 discusses communication and health teaching techniques as related to children, beginning with an overview of nursing process specific to communication with children. Types of learning, the influence of age on learning, and techniques for developing and implementing a teaching plan are included. Health teaching for a surgical experience is used as an example.

LEARNING OBJECTIVES

After mastering the content in this chapter, you should be able to do the following:

1. Describe the principles of effective communication and teaching and learning as they relate to health teaching with children.
2. Assess children for their ability to communicate and readiness to learn.
3. State nursing diagnoses related to communication and health teaching with children.
4. Identify expected outcomes for a specific child based on the child's age, developmental maturity, emotional needs, and communication or learning style.
5. Plan nursing care based on the use of communication and health teaching priorities.
6. Implement health teaching (e.g., devising a puppet show) using principles of effective communication and teaching–learning.
7. Evaluate outcome criteria to be certain that outcomes established for care have been achieved.
8. Identify National Health Goals related to communicating with and teaching children that nurses could be instrumental in helping the nation achieve.
9. Identify areas of care related to effective communication or health teaching of children that could benefit from additional nursing research or application of evidence-based nursing practice.
10. Use critical thinking to analyze ways that therapeutic communication and health teaching can be further incorporated into the nursing care of children and families.
11. Integrate knowledge of effective communication and teaching–learning with the nursing process to achieve quality maternal and child health nursing care.

KEY TERMS

affective learning
behavior modification
clarifying
cognitive learning
communication
demonstration
empathy
feedback
focusing
health fairs
nontherapeutic communication
paraphrasing
perception checking
positive reinforcement
psychomotor learning
redemonstration
reflecting
teaching plan
therapeutic communication

■ Mastering the Information

MATCHING

Match the terms in Column I with a definition, example, or related statement from Column II. Place the letter corresponding to the answer in the space provided.

COLUMN I

1. _____Nontherapeutic communication
2. _____Therapeutic communication
3. _____Feedback
4. _____Reflecting
5. _____Clarifying
6. _____Perception checking

7. _____Focusing
8. _____Paraphrasing

COLUMN II

a. Helping someone center on a subject that you suspect is causing anxiety because he or she comments about it indirectly or completely avoids it
b. Interaction that is planned, has structure, and is helpful and constructive
c. Repeating statements someone has made so that you both can be certain you understood
d. Restating the last word or phrase someone has said when there is a pause in the communication
e. Documenting a feeling or emotion that someone has expressed to you
f. Restating what someone has said not only to indicate that you have heard correctly but to help explain what the person is trying to say
g. Interaction that lacks structure, planning, and deliberate purpose
h. A response acknowledging a message has been received and understood

COLUMN I

1. ____Behavior modification
2. ____Cognitive learning
3. ____Informal teaching
4. ____Learning
5. ____Lifestyle
6. ____Psychomotor learning
7. ____Puppetry
8. ____Resource people
9. ____Role modeling
10. ____Teaching
11. ____Affective learning

COLUMN II

A. A two-step process involving the acquisition of knowledge and resulting in a measurable change in behavior
B. Process that involves a change in an individual's ability to perform a skill
C. Process that involves a change in the individual's level of understanding or knowledge
D. Individuals specializing in teaching particular information or skills
E. A system aimed at erasing some form of activity that interferes with health functioning
F. Presentation of information so as to increase someone's knowledge or insight
G. The common pattern of a child's life
H. A helpful method for teaching preschool children about the hospital and health care staff
I. Process occurring when a nurse spontaneously answers a child's or parent's question about a care measure
J. Demonstration of a certain attitude that you want a child to learn
K. Process that involves a change in a person's attitude

SHORT ANSWER

Supply the missing term or the information requested.

1. ________ ________ is a method that examines statements, thoughts, and responses to determine effectiveness with therapeutic communication.
2. Teaching in the home gives the nurse an opportunity to assess the child's ________, interactions with ________ ________, and overall ________ ________________________.
3. Provide the term for the type of learning described. ________ depends on muscle and neurologic coordination. ________ requires adequate development, intelligence, and attention span. ________ is gained best through role modeling, role playing, or shared-experience discussion.
4. ______ ______ is exact imitation of a demonstrated procedure.
5. Learning goals should reflect the ________ of learning desired and should establish ________ and ________________ guidelines.
6. When teaching a psychomotor skill, always assess the child's ________ ________ to perform the procedure.
7. Discuss three benefits of group teaching.
8. Describe the first step in developing a teaching plan.
9. Discuss the benefit of using visual aids when teaching children.
10. Explain the concept of learning ability plateaus.

11. Discuss nursing measures that will help the nation achieve health goals related to communication and health teaching as an important mechanism of preventive health care.

CRITICAL EXPLORATION

Examine the discharge teaching forms or documentation at a local health care facility. Evaluate the clarity of instructions for children of various age groups.

■ Applying Your Knowledge

CASE STUDY

Six-year-old Raoul Mendelez has been newly diagnosed with diabetes. He understands both English and Spanish, although his parents communicate with him and each other almost exclusively in Spanish.

1. As the nurse caring for Raoul, what communication and teaching techniques will you use to maximize his and his parents' comprehension of the disease and the lifestyle changes it will necessitate?
2. During your first teaching session, you notice the parents are constantly interrupting and questioning Raoul, and they appear anxious. You realize you must modify your teaching plan to improve effectiveness. What adjustments would you make?
3. How might your teaching plan change if Raoul were 16 years old?
4. What effects might Raoul's Hispanic culture have on your communication and teaching plan?

CRITICAL INQUIRY EXERCISE

1. Prepare and execute a teaching plan for an adolescent and a school-age child on some aspect of health maintenance or health promotion. Evaluate the effectiveness of your communication and teaching and note the differences in approach and content needed for each group.
2. Prepare a teaching plan for a toddler related to nutrition. Use a creative approach and evaluate its effectiveness in helping the child learn the content presented.

■ Practicing for NCLEX

MULTIPLE-CHOICE QUESTIONS

Circle the letter that corresponds to the best answer for each question.

1. Which of the following indicates appropriate use of teaching–learning principles?
   A. Explaining to a school-age child that the kidney transplant is being done because it will be good for him
   B. Providing a booklet that encourages a preschool child to eat extra meat because it will help to repair his incision
   C. Having the mother of an infant use a game to teach the infant a desired activity
   D. Using a firm tone to tell a toddler not to touch her bandage
2. A child may have the greatest difficulty learning which of the following?
   A. Dietary adjustments
   B. Insulin administration
   C. Colostomy irrigation
   D. Range-of-motion exercises
3. Which of the following is true about children relative to learning?
   A. One child's learning style may differ from another's.
   B. Admitting your discomfort with teaching a subject will negatively affect learning.
   C. Chronologic age is more indicative of learning capability than mental age.
   D. The older the child, the shorter the attention span.
4. Sally has to teach a group of preschoolers to dial 911. The most effective strategy for this teaching would be:
   A. Pamphlets
   B. Lecture
   C. Discussion
   D. Demonstration

5. Which of the following should be included in the teaching–learning process with a young child?
   A. Focusing information solely to the child, since parents cannot change the child's behavior
   B. Evaluating if the child is performing the desired behavior when indicated
   C. Letting the child decide the depth of information to be taught
   D. Teaching the child special ways to prepare the food on a restricted diet

ALTERNATE FORMAT QUESTIONS

Fill in the Blank

Supply the missing term or the information requested.

1. Teaching strategies are most effective when they are ______________________________.
2. The use of flash cards or board games may assist a child in ______________ certain information.
3. Since children often absorb one piece of information at a time, preparation for surgery should be taught in ______________________________.
4. Children learn best those things that hold a particular ______________________ for them.
5. Learning occurs best with ______ reinforcement.

Multiple-Answer Multiple Choice

Circle the letter(s) corresponding to the appropriate answer(s). Select all that apply.

1. Which of the following nursing interventions are appropriate?
   A. Provide a long, clear explanation about procedures to preschool clients to facilitate understanding.
   B. Have parents present each time health teaching is performed with adolescents.
   C. Offer an immediate, concrete reward to school-age children to encourage learning.
   D. Assess the child's family patterns before planning the timing for exercise or medication activities after discharge.
   E. Avoid using puppets for teaching preschool children.
   F. Teach multiple ways of performing a skill the first time you teach the skill.
   G. Correct a wrong action by first acknowledging a positive aspect of what the child did or how the child performed the action.

UNIT VII

The Nursing Role in Supporting the Health of Ill Children and Their Families

CHAPTER 35

Nursing Care of the Ill Child and Family

CHAPTER OVERVIEW

Chapter 35 provides an overview of the experience of hospitalization and its effect on children from infancy through adolescence and their families. The meaning of the hospital experience to children is discussed. The role of play therapy in the preparation and care of the hospitalized child is reviewed. The use of the nursing process to plan and provide care for the hospitalized child and the family is reviewed.

LEARNING OBJECTIVES

After mastering the content in this chapter, you should be able to do the following:

1. Describe the meaning of illness and home care, ambulatory, and in-hospital experiences to children.
2. Assess the impact of an illness, especially one requiring a hospital stay, on a child.
3. Formulate nursing diagnoses related to the stress of illness in children.
4. Establish appropriate outcomes for the ill child.
5. Plan nursing care to reduce the stress of illness, such as helping parents plan for hospitalization or home care.
6. Implement measures such as orientation, education, and therapeutic play to reduce the stress of illness.
7. Evaluate outcomes for achievement and effectiveness of care for the ill child.
8. Identify National Health Goals related to hospitalization or health care that nurses can be instrumental in helping the nation achieve.
9. Identify areas related to illness in children that could benefit from additional nursing research or application of evidence-based practice.
10. Use critical thinking to analyze ways in which illness can be made more family-centered and less traumatic for children.
11. Integrate knowledge about the child's response to illness with the nursing process to achieve quality maternal and child health nursing care.

KEY TERMS

case management nursing
calorie counting
direct care
home care
hospice care
indirect care
non-rapid-eye movement (NREM) sleep
play therapy
primary nursing
rapid-eye movement (REM) sleep
sensory overload
skilled home care
sleep deprivation
therapeutic play

■ Mastering the Information

MATCHING

Match the terms in Column I with a definition, example, or related statement from Column II. Place the letter corresponding to the answer in the space provided.

COLUMN I

1. _____Observation play
2. _____Cooperative play
3. _____Creative play
4. _____Dramatic play
5. _____Parallel play
6. _____Play
7. _____Play therapy
8. _____Therapeutic play

COLUMN II

a. A psychoanalytic technique used by psychiatrists to help children understand their feelings, thoughts, and motives
b. A play technique that is divided into three parts: energy release, dramatic play, and creative play
c. The "work" of children: a means by which children develop increasing cognitive, psychomotor, and social capabilities

d. Acting out an anxiety situation; most effective with preschoolers
e. Type of play in which children watch play intently but are not actively engaged in it
f. Two children playing side by side but seldom attempting to interact with each other
g. Children playing with an organized structure or competing for a desired goal or outcome
h. The child's drawing a picture or making a list to express emotions or knowledge level

TRUE OR FALSE

Indicate if the following statements are true or false by placing a "T" or "F" in the space provided.

______ 1. Children are not just small adults.

______ 2. Children should be told that the doctor will be "taking their tonsils out."

______ 3. New foods should be introduced to the hospitalized infant to promote growth and development.

______ 4. School-age children cannot describe symptoms with accuracy.

______ 5. Children can be reliable for monitoring their own care and speaking up about incorrect procedures and medications.

______ 6. Children need more nutrients than adults, and thus may require hospitalization for vomiting or diarrhea when adults would not.

______ 7. Children tend to respond to disease locally rather than systemically.

______ 8. Assess patient needs relative to cultural differences by using textbook descriptions of the needs of persons of that culture.

______ 9. Separation is most damaging to a child between ages 2 months and 3 months.

______10. Children older than age 7 should be told of a pending hospitalization as soon as the parents are aware of it.

SHORT ANSWER

Supply the missing term or the information requested.

1. The way children deal with hospitalization is based on the following factors: ——— of the event, ——— ——— available, and effectiveness of past ———————————————.
2. List five hazards common to all hospitalizations regardless of the reason or length of stay.
3. The response of children to illness depends on their ——— ———, past ———, and level of ———————————————.
4. Nurses can help the nation meet health care goals related to mental health of children by helping with assessment of children's ———level and reducing the ———of the hospitalization.
5. Parents of infants who will be hospitalized should bring the child's ——— ——— with the child to the hospital.
6. The three chief fears of the hospitalized toddler or preschooler are fear of the ———, ———, and ———————————————.
7. The school-age child and adolescent should have ——— explanations of what will happen in the hospital.
8. Describe why explanations of procedures to young children are not always successful in relieving the stress of illness and hospitalization.

■ Applying Your Knowledge

CASE STUDY

Devon, a 3-year-old who had emergency surgery while on vacation, has been separated from her single mother, who had to return home because of her job, and 14-year-old sister. Devon has been without her family for 4 days.

1. What behaviors would you expect Devon to display to nursing staff over the next days?
2. What effect might Devon's hospitalization and absence have on her mother and older sister?
3. What interventions might you plan for Devon and her family?

CRITICAL INQUIRY EXERCISE

1. What measures would you take to prepare a 4-month-old infant and family members for open heart surgery? How would this preparation differ if the surgery were minor?

2. Design a teaching plan for parents whose 2-year-old child will be admitted to the hospital for surgery.

CRITICAL EXPLORATION

1. While on a pediatric clinical unit, assess children in varying age groups. Determine if separation anxiety is present, and note the age levels of the children experiencing the highest levels of anxiety.

2. Interview the parent of a hospitalized child. Determine the type of preparation the parent used before bringing the child to the hospital.

■ Practicing for NCLEX

MULTIPLE-CHOICE QUESTIONS

Circle the letter that corresponds to the best answer for each question.

1. A 6-year-old is to be admitted to the hospital for an elective surgery. The nurse should advise the parents to tell the child about the surgery how many days before admission to prevent unnecessary worry?
   A. 1
   B. 2
   C. 4
   D. 6

2. The nurse might initiate which of the following interventions when caring for a hospitalized child with a disability or chronic illness?
   A. Avoid using information from previous hospitalizations when planning to prepare the child for the current hospitalization.
   B. Help the child avoid contact with peers while hospitalized to decrease self-consciousness and the sense of being different.
   C. Limit visiting hours to prevent fatigue of the child.
   D. Suggest the child write letters to friends or call family members.

3. Alice, age 2 years, is in the intensive care unit with multiple tubes and bandages. Her parents are present frequently but appear reluctant to handle Alice's tubes and bandages, although they asked to feed her at meals. The nurse should do which of the following?
   A. Inform the parents that it is important that they learn to change Alice's dressings and perform this procedure often.
   B. Encourage the parents to irrigate Alice's tubing to make them feel more involved in her plan of care.
   C. Allow the parents to feed Alice and do other care measures as they express interest and comfort.
   D. Limit the parents from performing any care for Alice so they will understand that nurses are capable of fully caring for her.

4. When preparing a child for procedures or surgery, the nurse might do which of the following?
   A. Instruct the child to place the thermometer into his or her arms and hold it there.
   B. Prepare the child for surgery by providing the child with a doll and a small scalpel.
   C. Provide a doll and syringe, alcohol wipes, and a tourniquet to prepare the child for a blood-drawing procedure.
   D. To help a child cope with a dressing change, allow the child to hand the sterile gauze to the nurse during the procedure.

5. Which of the following would be an appropriate method for influencing a child to assist with a care measure?
   A. Encourage fluid intake by explaining to the child that fluid will keep him from drying up.
   B. Have the child lift hand weights every 2 hours to strengthen muscles.
   C. Create board games and crossword puzzles to help the child learn about health teaching.
   D. Place an incentive spirometry machine in front of the child and instruct him or her in deep breathing.

ALTERNATE FORMAT QUESTIONS

Fill in the Blank

Supply the missing term or the information requested.

1. ——— is one of the most powerful tools available to the nurse in working toward the objective of a successful experience for the hospitalized child.
2. Determine the appropriate age range for the following childhood play activities.
   A. ——— Need toys in their cribs such as mobiles
   B. ——— Would enjoy watching a soap opera and then discussing the people and their problems
   C. ——— Need put-in and take-out toys, such as blocks that can be stacked
   D. ——— Need quiet toys such as crayons, markers, or books
3. Determine the child's symptoms as much by ——————— as by the child's report.

Multiple-Answer Multiple Choice

Circle the letter(s) corresponding to the appropriate answer(s). Select all that apply.

1. Which of the following nursing interventions are appropriate?
   A. Say grace before administering a tube feeding if the child commonly says grace before meals.
   B. Stand close to the child, at full adult height, during admission to establish a rapport with the child.
   C. Call the child "sugar" or "sweetie" when addressing him/her to create a warm environment and close relationship.
   D. Determine the child's routines and attempt to adapt the hospital routine as much as possible.
   E. Let the child wear his or her own clothes if possible rather than change to a hospital gown.
   F. Limit the number of readmissions and length of stay by teaching parents how to safely monitor their child after a procedure.
   G. Encourage younger siblings to visit, as well as siblings over the age of 12 or 14 years.
   H. Use a team nursing approach to provide the child with a variety of caregivers.
   I. Perform procedures such as blood drawing at the bedside to establish this area as the child's care area.
   J. Allow the child to make as many decisions during a procedure as possible to facilitate a sense of control.

CHAPTER 36

Nursing Care of the Child Undergoing Diagnostic Techniques and Other Therapeutic Modalities

CHAPTER OVERVIEW

Chapter 36 provides an overview of the nursing care required for the ill child and family during diagnostic and therapeutic procedures. Adaptations required for children when undergoing diagnostic procedures and various therapeutic techniques are discussed. The use of the nursing process to plan and provide care for the hospitalized child and the family is explored.

LEARNING OBJECTIVES

After mastering the content in this chapter, you should be able to do the following:

1. Describe common nursing interventions used in the health care of children to aid diagnosis and therapy.
2. Assess children as to developmental stage and knowledge level before beginning diagnostic or therapeutic procedures or other nursing interventions.
3. Formulate nursing diagnoses related to common diagnostic or therapeutic procedures used with children.
4. Identify outcomes for the child undergoing a diagnostic or therapeutic procedure.
5. Plan nursing interventions to aid in diagnosis or therapy for children.
6. Implement nursing interventions relevant to diagnostic or therapeutic procedures.
7. Evaluate outcomes related to diagnostic and therapeutic procedures for achievement.
8. Identify National Health Goals related to diagnostic and therapeutic procedures for children that nurses could be instrumental in helping the nation achieve.
9. Identify areas related to nursing procedures with children that could benefit from additional nursing research or application of evidence-based practice.
10. Use critical thinking to analyze ways that diagnostic and therapeutic procedures can be modified to meet the needs of children.
11. Integrate knowledge of common diagnostic and therapeutic procedures with the nursing process to achieve quality maternal and child health nursing.

KEY TERMS

aspiration studies
barium contrast studies
bronchoscopy
clean-catch urine specimen
colonoscopy
computed tomography (CT)
electrical impulse studies
endoscopy
gavage feedings
magnetic resonance imaging (MRI)
positron emission tomography (PET)
radiopharmaceutical
single photon emission computerized tomography (SPECT)
total parenteral nutrition (TPN)
ultrasound

■ Mastering the Information

MATCHING

Match the terms in Column I with a definition, example, or related statement from Column II. Place the letter corresponding to the answer in the space provided.

COLUMN I

1. _____Barium contrast studies
2. _____Gavage feedings
3. _____Total parenteral nutrition (TPN)
4. _____Bronchoscopy
5. _____Radiopharmaceutical

COLUMN II

a. Infusion of a concentrated hypertonic solution into a central or peripheral intravenous site
b. Radioactive-combined substances that when given orally or by injection flow to designated body organs for a diagnostic picture
c. Direct visualization of the larynx, trachea, and bronchi through a fiberoptic tube
d. Use of radiopaque dye to outline the gastrointestinal tract
e. Provision of adequate nutrition through a nasogastric tube

SHORT ANSWER

Supply the missing term or the information requested.

1. A ______-______ specimen involves collecting urine during usual voiding after the external meatus has been cleaned.
2. Two problems when using an ostomy appliance with an infant are ——— and ——— ———.
3. Discuss the psychological and physical preparation needed for a child undergoing surgery.
4. List four common types of restraints used with children.
5. Describe two ways in which nurses can help the nation achieve goals related to reducing the length of hospital stay for children.

■ Applying Your Knowledge

CASE STUDY

Iesha Jackson, age 2, is admitted to your care after stabilization of a sickle cell crisis. She is screaming for her mother and trying to get out of bed. Her mother, age 18, is in the waiting room making a call. She says Iesha's father is the custodial parent and this crisis happened on "her weekend" with Iesha. She doesn't want to call Iesha's father for fear he will blame her.

1. Iesha will require several invasive procedures during her stay. What teaching responsibilities do you have in this situation?
2. How will the fact that Iesha's parents are separated affect your discharge teaching plan?

CRITICAL INQUIRY EXERCISE

1. Review five skills listed in a fundamentals text that were not discussed in this chapter, and note ways in which those skills might need to be adjusted for an infant or child.
2. Plan a schedule for a 4-year-old child who must have blood drawn for lab work, an abdominal x-ray, a CT scan, and an endoscopy during her 2-day hospital stay.

CRITICAL EXPLORATION

Tour a pediatric unit and observe the procedures being performed. Compare the techniques used with those noted on an adult floor, and note any variations.

■ Practicing for NCLEX

MULTIPLE-CHOICE QUESTIONS

Circle the letter that corresponds to the best answer for each question.

1. When a procedure is being performed that requires a consent form, which of the following is true?
   A. A consent form can be omitted if the procedure involves only a minimal risk.
   B. The nurse must explain the procedure and obtain signed consent if the physician does not.
   C. Emancipated minors must have parental permission to sign a consent form.
   D. In single-parent families, the custodial parent must sign the consent form.

2. The nurse's role in assisting with diagnostic procedures includes which of the following?
   a. Helping the child to forget the experience of the procedure as quickly as possible
   b. Using complex medical terms to explain procedures to children and parents to demonstrate knowledge and competence
   c. Explaining the preparation and actual procedure before beginning either
   d. Sending mature children to different test departments without supervision to increase independence

3. Which of the following is appropriate when modifying procedures for children?
   a. Parents should be asked to restrain infants when indicated.
   b. Toddlers should be given procedures quickly and without warning to decrease resistance.
   c. Adolescents should be expected to tolerate procedures maturely and without fear.
   d. School-age children should be given an explanation of the reasons for procedures.

4. When performing contrast dye studies with children, the nurse should:
   a. Tell the child the flavored barium will taste like a milkshake to increase cooperation
   b. Isolate the child after the test until the radioactivity resolves
   c. Explain to the child that a warm feeling may be experienced with IV dye
   d. Restrict all activity for the duration of the procedure to prevent distracting the child

5. When teaching parents about temperature reduction in children, the nurse should include which of the following interventions?
   a. Administer acetylsalicylic acid every 4 hours until the child's temperature is less than 101°F.
   b. Dress the child in warm flannel night clothes to prevent chilling.
   c. Give the age-appropriate dose of ibuprofen (Motrin) to reduce temperature.
   d. Place an ice cloth on the child's forehead and refresh it every hour.

ALTERNATE FORMAT QUESTIONS

Fill in the Blank

Supply the missing term or the information requested.

1. Restraints should be checked every ——— minutes to ensure that circulation is intact.
2. When securing a dressing on infants and young children, use ——— tape.

Multiple-Answer Multiple Choice

Circle the letter(s) corresponding to the appropriate answer(s). Select all that apply.

1. Which of the following intervention(s) are appropriate?
   A. Allowing the child to look at the incision during a dressing change
   B. Taking a radial pulse for children under 1 year of age
   C. Ensuring that an infant is calm before assessing respiratory rate
   D. Taking an axillary or tympanic temperature in children from infancy to age 4
   E. Assessing blood pressure in routine assessment of children over 3 years of age
   F. Recognizing that in children it is normal to have a thigh blood pressure lower than the blood pressure in the arms
   G. Drawing a child's blood at the bedside to decrease the trauma of the experience
   H. Attaching a collection bag to a child who has not been toilet-trained to collect a urine specimen
   I. Pushing children to drink several glasses of fluid before voiding for a urine specimen
   J. Sponging children with cold water to lower the temperature
   K. Explaining to a school-age child that an ultrasound will be painful but is a necessary diagnostic procedure
   L. Telling a preschool child a shot will hurt but for only a short time
   M. Praising a child for cooperation even if none was visibly obvious
   N. Instructing adolescents on the cleaning procedure for clean-catch specimens

2. After an upper gastrointestinal endoscopy study, which of the following interventions would be important?
   A. Check for gag reflex before giving any oral fluids.
   B. Monitor airway and respiratory function for the first 4 hours.
   C. Apply a warm compress to the neck to reduce spasm.
   D. Administer atropine to reduce pulmonary secretions.
   E. Verify allergy to iodine or shellfish.

CHAPTER 37

Nursing Care of the Child Undergoing Medication Administration and Intravenous Therapy

CHAPTER OVERVIEW

Chapter 37 provides an overview of the nursing care required for the ill child and family regarding medication administration and intravenous therapy. Adaptations required for children during the preparation and administration of medications and when planning and implementing intravenous therapy are discussed. The use of the nursing process to plan and provide care for the child and the family involved in medication administration and intravenous therapy is explored.

LEARNING OBJECTIVES

After mastering the content in this chapter, you should be able to do the following:

1. Describe common methods of medication administration used in the health care of children.
2. Assess the developmental stage and knowledge level of children and adolescents before beginning medication administration.
3. Formulate nursing diagnoses related to medication administration with children.
4. Identify outcomes for children receiving medication.
5. Plan nursing interventions to aid in making medicine administration maximally effective.
6. Implement nursing interventions concerned with medication administration and children.
7. Evaluate outcomes related to medication administration with children.
8. Identify National Health Goals related to medication administration that nurses could be instrumental in helping the nation achieve.
9. Identify areas related to medication administration with children that could benefit from additional nursing research or application of evidence-based practice.
10. Use critical thinking to analyze ways that medication administration can be modified to meet the needs of children of all ages.
11. Integrate knowledge of medication administration with the nursing process to achieve quality maternal and child health nursing.

KEY TERMS

absorption
distribution
excretion
Intracath
intermittent infusion devices
metabolism
pharmacokinetics
vascular access port

■ Mastering the Information

MATCHING

Match the terms in Column I with a definition, example, or related statement from Column II. Place the letter corresponding to the answer in the space provided.

COLUMN I

1. _____Absorption
2. _____Distribution
3. _____Excretion
4. _____Metabolism
5. _____Pharmacokinetics

COLUMN II

a. Removal of the drug or metabolites from the body to prevent drug toxicity
b. Process that determines the intensity and duration of a drug's action
c. Conversion of the drug into an active form or an inactive form

d. Movement of the drug through the bloodstream to a specific site of action

e. Transfer of the drug from its point of entry into the bloodstream

SHORT ANSWER

Supply the missing term or the information requested.

1. Identify four routes by which medications are given to children.
2. Before administering any medication to a child, confirm that the dose ordered is correct for the child's ——— or ——— ———.
3. A ——— ——— ——— can be used to draw frequent venous blood samples.
4. Discuss how age may alter drug absorption, distribution, inactivation, and excretion.
5. Explain circumstances under which restraints may be used with infants and children during intravenous therapy.
6. List three fluid infusion safety measures to be used with children.
7. The six rights of medication administration are Right ———, ———, ———, ———, ———, and ———.

■ Applying Your Knowledge

CASE STUDY

India Jeilhal is admitted to your care after a playground accident. The 5-year-old is sitting up in bed holding her mother's hand. The doctor has ordered an IV to infuse an antibiotic as well as oral pain medication. India's mother is asking you to give India something for pain.

1. How would you respond to India's mother's request? What teaching responsibilities do you have in this situation?
2. How will you prepare for the initiation of intravenous therapy? What measures will you take to prepare India and her mother for the procedure?

CRITICAL INQUIRY EXERCISE

1. Discuss ways in which you might need to alter your approach when administering an intramuscular injection to a 1-month-old, a 1-year-old, a 5-year-old, a 10-year-old, or a 16-year-old child.
2. Plan instructions for the parents of a 4-year-old child who must administer an oral medication that comes in tablet form only.

CRITICAL EXPLORATION

Tour a neonatal unit and pediatric unit and observe intravenous therapy in place with children of various ages. Compare the techniques and equipment used with the different age groups.

■ Practicing for NCLEX

MULTIPLE-CHOICE QUESTIONS

Circle the letter that corresponds to the best answer for each question.

1. Sites frequently used for intravenous insertion in young children or infants include which of the following?
   A. Antecubital and veins on the extensor surface of the wrist
   B. Jugular and veins on the ventral surface of the hand
   C. Veins located in the leg or on the surface of the foot
   D. Radial or ulnar surface veins or the subclavian vein
2. The nurse preparing to initiate intravenous therapy with a 1-year-old infant would obtain which of the following size catheters?
   A. 16-gauge
   B. 18-gauge
   C. 20-gauge
   D. 22-gauge

3. A child weighing 20 kg is to begin fluid therapy. Based on caloric expenditure per 24 hours, the child should receive how many milliliters of maintenance intravenous solution?
   A. 1,500
   B. 1,725
   C. 2,000
   D. 2,300

4. The nurse can be instrumental in helping the nation achieve national health goals related to children and drugs or medication administration by:
   A. Stressing the importance of using medications to treat every discomfort
   B. Educating parents regarding the importance of steroid use to treat acne in adolescents
   C. Teaching stress management techniques to children and parents for use to address anxiety
   D. Instructing parents to keep medication at the bedside for ease of access

5. A 3-year-old child may receive a medication dosage consistent with the dosage usually given to a 1-year-old if the 3-year-old child:
   A. Was developmentally delayed
   B. Was tall for his/her age
   C. Had the body surface area of a 1-year-old
   D. Weighed more than a 1-year-old

6. When assessing a child before medication administration, it is important to determine which of the following?
   A. The child's dosage preference
   B. Past medication-taking experiences
   C. Parental developmental status
   D. Whether the medication is having the desired effect

ALTERNATE FORMAT QUESTIONS

Fill in the Blank

Supply the missing term or the information requested.

1. When administering nose drops, place the child on his or her ———.
2. The mandatory site for intramuscular injections in infants is the ——— ———.
3. ——— therapy is the quickest and most effective means of administering fluid or medicine to the ill infant or child.
4. The ——— of body systems in infants and children plays a major role in drug action.
5. To administer ear drops to a child under 2 years, straighten the ear canal by pulling the pinna ——— and ———.

Multiple-Answer Multiple Choice

Circle the letter(s) corresponding to the appropriate answer(s). Select all that apply.

1. Select the appropriate intervention(s) for a child who is to receive oral medication therapy.
   A. Instruct parents to store drugs in locked, elevated cabinets.
   B. Ask a child, "Will you drink this for me?" to help the child feel respected.
   C. Tell the child it is time to take the medicine and asking the child's preference of fluid to take the medicine with.
   D. Mix bitter medicine with a full glass of juice to dilute the taste.
   E. Crush a tablet and mix it with applesauce for better taste when appropriate.

CHAPTER 38

Pain Management in Children

CHAPTER OVERVIEW

Chapter 38 discusses the management of pain in children. The causes of pain as well as the assessment and measurement of pain are discussed, with emphasis on developmental considerations. Varied pain management strategies are reviewed, including pharmacologic and nonpharmacologic measures. The use of the nursing process to plan and provide appropriate care and teaching to promote appropriate pain management in children is discussed.

LEARNING OBJECTIVES

After mastering the content in this chapter, you should be able to do the following:

1. Describe the major methods of pain management in children.
2. Use the nursing process to identify physical and psychological aspects of care required for the child who is in pain and to plan and implement that care.
3. Identify National Health Goals related to children with pain that nurses could be instrumental in helping the nation achieve.
4. Use critical thinking to analyze ways that nursing care for a child with pain could be more family-centered.
5. Integrate knowledge of pain in children with the nursing process to achieve quality child health nursing care.

KEY TERMS

acute pain
chronic pain
conscious sedation
distraction
epidural analgesia
gate control theory
imagery
pain
pain threshold
patient-controlled analgesia
referred pain
substitution of meaning
thought stopping
transcutaneous electrical nerve stimulation

■ Mastering the Information

MATCHING

Match the terms in Column I with a definition, example, or related statement from Column II. Place the letter corresponding to the answer in the space provided.

COLUMN I

1. _____Distraction
2. _____Gate control theory
3. _____Patient-controlled analgesia
4. _____Thought stopping
5. _____Transcutaneous electrical nerve stimulation

COLUMN II

a. A technique whereby children are taught to substitute a positive or relaxing thought for anxious thoughts

b. Use of a current to interfere with the transmission of the pain impulse across small nerve fibers

c. Explanation of pain impulses traveling between a site of injury and the brain, where the impulse is actually registered as pain

d. Cells of the brain stem that register an impulse as pain becoming preoccupied with other stimuli so the pain impulse cannot register

e. Self-administering of intravenous opiate boluses with a medication pump to control pain

SHORT ANSWER

Supply the missing term or the information requested.

1. The technique that allows the child to be both pain-free and sedated for a procedure and leaves protective reflexes intact is called ——— ———.
2. A numerical or ——— ——— scale uses a straight line with end points marked 0 for no pain on the left and 10 for worst pain on the right.

3. ——— ——— ——— or guided imagery is a distraction technique that helps a child place another, nonpainful meaning on a painful procedure.
4. Discuss two of three reasons that nurses do not provide adequate pain relief to children.
5. Explain why pain assessment might be difficult with children.
6. Briefly discuss the gate control theory.

■ Applying Your Knowledge

CASE STUDY

Patricia Walters, age 4, is admitted onto your unit after having her tonsils removed. Her mother is concerned that Patricia might have pain but says she is afraid of injections.

1. Patricia's mother asks if you will need to hold Patricia down because she hates needles but needs something for pain. What are some responses you might give?
2. What are some methods you might use to assess Patricia's pain? Which pain assessment tools would be inappropriate?

CRITICAL INQUIRY EXERCISE

1. What key points would you address in a teaching plan for a school-age child and parents when the child is discharged home after a painful day surgery? In addition to pain medication, what other pain relief measures might you include in this teaching plan?
2. What should you do if a school-age child or adolescent who is 1 day post surgery and has had no pain medication since surgery denies pain but shows signs of discomfort?

CRITICAL EXPLORATION

Visit a pediatric cancer unit and a postoperative inpatient care unit at a pediatric hospital. Compare the pain control methods used on each unit. Note the route of administration and the types of analgesics used.

■ Practicing for NCLEX

MULTIPLE-CHOICE QUESTIONS

Circle the letter that corresponds to the best answer for each question.

1. When assessing the pain of an infant, the nurse should consider which of the following?
   A. Infants are preverbal, so cues such as tears or guarding a body part can be helpful.
   B. Infants can be comforted completely by a parent if the pain is very intense.
   C. An infant can indicate if he or she has pain and exactly where the pain is located.
   D. Since infants think concretely, they may associate words like "sharp" with knives.
2. Which of the following is true about pain assessment for the school-age child and adolescent?
   A. A scale of 1 to 10 should be used for younger children to provide the child with maximum choices.
   B. Some children may require preassessment work to evaluate if they understand incremental measurements.
   C. School-age children use mechanisms for controlling pain that are unique and different from adult mechanisms.
   D. Preadolescents think very concretely, so they can describe pain with little difficulty.
3. Which of the following tools allows the health care provider to rate pain without the need of self-report input by the child and evaluates behaviors usually seen with pain?
   A. Logs and diaries of pain episodes
   B. "Oucher" pain rating scale
   C. FLACC pain assessment tool
   D. Poker chip tool

4. Analgesia instilled in the space just outside the spinal canal is called:
   A. Local anesthesia
   B. Epidural analgesia
   C. Intranasal analgesia
   D. Intravenous analgesia

ALTERNATE FORMAT QUESTIONS

Fill in the Blank

Supply the missing term or the information requested.

1. To reduce the pain of procedures such as venipuncture or lumbar puncture, a ——— ——— cream may be applied.

2. ——— ——— is an advantageous and cost-effective pharmacologic pain control method that is relatively easy to administer.

Multiple-Answer Multiple Choice

1. When preparing a teaching plan about the physiology of pain, the nurse includes the following events. Place these events in the proper sequence from first to last.
   A. Pain impulse perceived as pain
   B. Pain stimulus occurs
   C. Activation of nociceptors
   D. Interpretation of the sensation by the brain
   E. Sensation is routed to the spinal cord

UNIT VIII

The Nursing Role in Restoring and Maintaining the Health of Children and Families With Physiologic Disorders

CHAPTER 39

Nursing Care of the Child Born With a Physical Developmental Disorder

CHAPTER OVERVIEW

Chapter 39 reviews several defects seen among children and examines nursing strategies and implementations used during therapy and corrective and surgical procedures. This chapter also assists students in synthesizing the knowledge needed to formulate appropriate nursing care plans and evaluate the outcome of nursing goals for children with physical developmental disorders. A case study guides the student in assessing and determining proper nursing interventions for a client with a spinal and neurologic defect.

LEARNING OBJECTIVES

After mastering the content in this chapter, you should be able to do the following:

1. Describe common physical developmental birth disorders.
2. Assess a newborn who is born physically challenged.
3. Develop nursing diagnoses for the child with a physical developmental disorder.
4. Establish outcomes to meet the needs of the child with a physical developmental disorder.
5. Plan nursing care to meet the established outcomes of care for the child born with a physical developmental disorder.
6. Carry out nursing interventions for care of children born with physical developmental disorders, such as preventing infection in the child with spina bifida.
7. Evaluate outcomes to determine achievement and effectiveness of care.
8. Identify National Health Goals related to children born with physical disabilities that nurses could be instrumental in helping the nation achieve.
9. Identify areas related to developmentally challenged infants that could benefit by additional nursing research or application of evidence-based practice.
10. Use critical thinking to analyze the impact of a developmentally challenged child on the family and propose ways to make care more family-centered.
11. Integrate knowledge of congenital physical anomalies with the nursing process to achieve quality maternal and child health nursing care.

KEY TERMS

ankyloglossia
atresia
cleft lip
cleft palate
developmental hip dysplasia
fistula
frenulum
hydrocephalus
meconium plug
omphalocele
polydactyly
spina bifida
stenosis
syndactyly
transillumination
volvulus

■ Mastering the Information

MATCHING

Match the terms in Column I with a definition, example, or related statement from Column II. Place the letter corresponding to the answer in the space provided.

COLUMN I

1. ____Ankyloglossia
2. ____Pierre Robin syndrome
3. ____Diaphragmatic hernia
4. ____Torticollis

5. ____Meconium ileus
6. ____Hydrocephalus
7. ____Craniosynostosis
8. ____Thyroglossal cyst
9. ____Polydactyly
10. ____Umbilical hernia
11. ____Talipes
12. ____Achondroplasia
13. ____Microcephaly
14. ____Atresia
15. ____Gastroschisis
16. ____Fistula
17. ____Frenulum
18. ____Pectus excavatum

COLUMN II

a. Slow brain growth resulting in mental retardation
b. Occurs almost exclusively in newborns who are later diagnosed with cystic fibrosis due to absent enzyme
c. Defect arising from an embryogenic fault leaving a growth at the base of the tongue that drains through a fistula
d. Protrusion of abdominal organs into the chest cavity through a defect in the diaphragm
e. Restriction of the tongue caused by an abnormally tight frenulum
f. Birth defect identified as a trait anomaly: small mandible, cleft palate, and glossoptosis
g. Defect in cartilage production resulting in stunted growth of arms and legs
h. Protrusion of a portion of the intestine through umbilical ring, muscle, fascia
i. One or more additional fingers
j. Ankle-foot deformity
k. Injury to sternocleidomastoid muscle during birth, resulting in infant holding head tilted to the side
l. Premature closure of sutures of the skull
m. Indentation of the lower portion of the sternum, decreasing lung volume and displacing the heart to the left
n. Opening in the esophagus leading to the trachea
o. Membrane attached to lower anterior tip of tongue
p. Complete closure, such as due to absence of canalization in the bowel
q. Excess of cerebrospinal fluid in the ventricles and subarachnoid spaces of the brain
r. Herniation of abdominal contents without peritoneal membrane to contain it

SHORT ANSWER

Supply the missing term or the information requested.

1. ——— ——— deformity is due to an overgrowth of the neural tube in the 16th to 20th week of fetal growth.
2. A ——— ——— is a hard portion of meconium completely obstructing the intestinal lumen.
3. ——— and ——— ——— are the two types of developmental hip dysplasia.

■ Applying Your Knowledge

CASE STUDY

Patrick is approximately 24 hours old. The doctors are implementing tests and procedures to determine if his congenital neural tube defect is a meningocele or a myelomeningocele.

1. How does a meningocele different from a myelomeningocele?
2. What are the physical characteristics that Patrick would exhibit if diagnosed with a myelomeningocele?
3. Preoperatively, Patrick should be placed in what position?
4. The nurse should give special attention to Patrick's elimination status. What procedure might the nurse implement to aid in bladder elimination?

CRITICAL INQUIRY EXERCISE

1. Create a teaching plan for parents to perform a neurologic assessment on a child discharged from the hospital in a spica cast.

2. Identify the major components of the assessment when examining an infant for a diaphragmatic hernia. What are the physiologic explanations for the positive findings that you might find on assessment?

CRITICAL EXPLORATION

1. Visit the physical therapy department at your clinical facility. Identify the equipment used for motor development by the patients in the hospital and by the patients who visit for outpatient therapy.

2. Visit a community agency that sponsors the annual Special Olympics in your area. Speak with an appropriate staff member to learn some basic psychosocial skills on how to communicate with and motivate the child who has a chronic physical developmental defect.

■ Practicing for NCLEX

MULTIPLE-CHOICE QUESTIONS

Circle the letter that corresponds to the best answer for each question.

1. Leonard, age 8 months, is visiting the health clinic for a well-baby check-up. He is diagnosed with developmental hip dysplasia. The physician describes the defect as no communication between the femoral head and the acetabulum. This dysplasia is called:
   A. Preluxation
   B. Subluxation
   C. Dislocation
   D. Acetabular subluxation

2. A nurse performing the assessment on an infant with hip dysplasia would find that the affected extremity:
   A. Appears slightly shorter than the normal one
   B. Is resistant to extension
   C. Will not allow the child to lie supine with feet flexed
   D. Is obviously malformed

3. Dayle is a 3-month-old admitted to the hospital with a diagnosis of hydrocephalus. Which of the following findings would the nurse interpret as least indicative of increased intracranial pressure?
   A. Overriding sutures
   B. Shrill cry
   C. Hyperactive reflexes
   D. Prominent scalp veins

4. After a shunt to relieve intracranial pressure, which of the following would lead the nurse to suspect an infection?
   A. Subnormal temperature
   B. Decreased pulse
   C. Marked irritability
   D. Flexible neck

5. Crying is to be avoided in a child who has had a cleft lip repair because it:
   A. Sustains a traumatic experience
   B. Places tension on the suture line
   C. Threatens maternal–infant bonding
   D. Predisposes to respiratory difficulties

6. After repair of a tracheoesophageal fistula, the nurse would watch the infant carefully at postoperative days 7 to 10 for which of the following that would indicate a leak at sites of anastomosis?
   A. Serous drainage
   B. Acute indigestion
   C. Profuse diarrhea
   D. Respiratory distress

ALTERNATE FORMAT QUESTIONS

Fill in the Blank

Supply the missing term or the information requested.

1. __________ is the absence of the cerebral hemisphere of the brain.
2. __________ is the audible noise heard when the femoral head dislocates from the acetabulum.

Multiple-Answer Multiple Choice

Circle the letter(s) corresponding to the appropriate answer(s). Select all that apply.

1. When caring for an infant with a meningocele preoperatively, the nurse should:
   A. Irrigate the back of the head with saline every 2 hours
   B. Place a rolled towel under the abdomen pillow under the infant's head
   C. Position the infant supine with the head of bed at 45 degrees
   D. Place a piece of plastic on the child's back below the meningocele
   E. Replace the wet compress every 4 hours with a fresh saline compress
2. Desmond is admitted to the surgical floor of the pediatric hospital several hours after birth for a tracheoesophageal fistula. Which of the following would the nurse expect to assess?
   A. Constantly blowing mucus bubbles from the mouth
   B. Absence of stools
   C. Absence of rooting reflex
   D. Inability to swallow
   E. Respiratory distress

CHAPTER 40

Nursing Care of the Child With a Respiratory Disorder

CHAPTER OVERVIEW

Respiratory diseases are serious in children because the lumens of respiratory structures are small in children and likely to become obstructed in disease. Nurses need good assessment skills to assess clinical status. This chapter presents the most common disorders of the upper and lower respiratory tract, along with their therapeutic management. Care that incorporates the provision of airway patency by administering aerosols and bronchodilators, postural drainage and position changes, and antibiotics for infection is also addressed.

LEARNING OBJECTIVES

After mastering the content in this chapter, you should be able to do the following:

1. Describe common respiratory illnesses in children.
2. Assess the child with a respiratory illness.
3. Use the nursing process to formulate and address nursing diagnoses related to respiratory illness in children.
4. Identify National Health Goals related to children with respiratory disorders that nurses could be instrumental in helping the nation achieve.
5. Identify areas related to care of children with respiratory disorders that could benefit from additional nursing research.
6. Use critical thinking to analyze ways that nursing care for a child with a respiratory illness could be more family-centered.
7. Synthesize knowledge of respiratory illness in children with the nursing process to achieve quality maternal and child health nursing care.

KEY TERMS

adventitious sounds
aspiration
atelectasis
bronchial breathing
clubbing
cupping
cyanosis
expiration
hypoxemia
hypoxia
inspiration
paroxysmal coughing
percussion
pneumothorax
postural drainage
rales
retraction
stridor
tachypnea
vesicular breathing
wheezing

■ Mastering the Information

MATCHING

Match the terms in Column I with a definition, example, or related statement from Column II. Place the letter corresponding to the answer in the space provided.

COLUMN I

1. ____Hypoxia
2. ____Dyspnea
3. ____Hypoventilation
4. ____Apnea
5. ____Hyperventilation
6. ____Anoxia
7. ____Tachypnea
8. ____Hypoxemia
9. ____Bronchopulmonary dysplasia
10. ____Laryngeal stridor
11. ____Rales
12. ____Wheezing

COLUMN II

a. Lack of respiration
b. Rapid deep breathing
c. Difficulty in respiratory exchange
d. Decreased oxygen in body cells
e. Reduction below adequate levels of oxygen in tissue
f. Rapid respiration
g. Deficit oxygen content in the blood
h. Shallow breathing
i. Fine crackling sounds
j. Harsh, high-pitched sound heard on inspiration
k. Chronic lung condition seen in infants with acute respiratory distress at birth
l. Expiratory whistling sound due to obstruction of lower trachea or bronchioles

SHORT ANSWER

Supply the missing term or the information requested.

1. The upper respiratory tract functions to ———, ——— , and ——— air.
2. Five common terms used to describe respiratory dysfunctions are ———, ———, ———, ———, and ———————————.
3. Identify the normal values for each of these blood gas components: Po_2 ——— ; PCO_2 ——— ; O_2 saturation ——— ; pH ——— ; HCO_3 ———.
4. The most dangerous periods following a tonsillectomy are the ——— , and days——— to ———.
5. If a child has no complications following a tonsillectomy, he or she is discharged the same day or the following morning. Three danger signs you would tell the parents to watch for are ———, ——————— , and ———————.
6. Children with symptoms of epiglottitis should never be examined with a tongue blade because the gagging might cause ——— ——— ———.
7. Three symptoms of epiglottitis are ———————, ——————— , and ———————.
8. Nurses can help the nation achieve health goals focused on respiratory illness in children by teaching children to avoid ——— ——— , by teaching programs to help children with asthma learn ways of ——— ——— and take steps to reduce the severity of an attack, and by encouraging parents to come for ——— ——— visits.

■ Applying Your Knowledge

CASE STUDY

Rebecca O'Shea is a 2-year-old with cystic fibrosis. Her mother is a working single parent. Rebecca was admitted to your unit with a diagnosis of pneumonia. Her mother expresses concern that Rebecca will die because working makes it difficult for her to perform the respiratory care Rebecca requires.

1. What are the major problems you would address for Rebecca during her hospital stay?
2. Your discharge plan would need to address what family needs?
3. How might community agencies be beneficial in assisting Rebecca and her mother?

CRITICAL INQUIRY EXERCISE

1. In what way, if any, would you need to alter your approach and process when practicing respiratory assessment on a child compared to an adult?
2. Develop a discharge teaching plan for parents of infants or children with an upper respiratory infection.

CRITICAL EXPLORATION

1. Spend a day at the cystic fibrosis clinic at a local hospital to observe follow-up care and treatment.
2. Spend a day with a respiratory therapist on a pediatric unit to observe various treatments and modalities.

■ Practicing for NCLEX

MULTIPLE-CHOICE QUESTIONS

Circle the letter that corresponds to the best answer for each question.

1. Which of the following actions would be most appropriate when assessing a newborn for choanal atresia?
   A. Make the newborn cry, and then gently compress one nostril and then the second.
   B. Compress both nostrils at the same time and open the newborn's mouth.
   C. Hold the newborn's mouth closed and then compress one nostril and then the second.
   D. Have the newborn suck on a bottle as you compress the nostrils.

2. Baby Jane was diagnosed with acute nasopharyngitis (common cold). Her mother is being taught how to use a bulb syringe and a vaporizer to clear the congestion. Which of the following would the nurse include in the teaching plan?
   A. The bulb should be compressed before inserting the syringe into the child's nostril.
   B. The vaporizer should be kept at the bedside so the mist will be close to the child's face.
   C. The vaporizer will not require cleaning since the steam is very hot and sterile.
   D. The bulb syringe should be filled with saline nose drops that should be squeezed into the nostril.

3. Baby John was admitted with streptococcal pharyngitis. When he was discharged, his mother was told to return to the doctor's office in 2 weeks with a urine specimen. The nurse understands that the rationale for this instruction is that the urine would be examined most likely:
   A. For fat and lipids to see if the kidneys are working
   B. For protein to determine if acute glomerulonephritis is developing
   C. To determine if the child is developing otitis media
   D. To determine whether or not to increase the child's diet from liquid to soft

4. Which of the following would be inappropriate to include in the plan of care for a child who has had a tonsillectomy?
   A. Observing for signs of bleeding
   B. Pushing ice cream hourly to soothe the child's throat
   C. Placing the child on his or her abdomen with a pillow under the chest
   D. Observing for excessive swallowing and throat clearing.

5. If bleeding occurs in a child following a tonsillectomy, the nursing action would be to:
   A. Elevate the child's head and turn him or her on his or her side
   B. Place the child in a prone position
   C. Place the child in a Trendelenburg position
   D. Elevate the child's feet and turn him or her in a prone position

6. Which of the following should be given to a child following a tonsillectomy?
   A. Sips of clear liquid or ice chips
   B. Milkshakes or scoops of ice cream
   C. French fries
   D. Popcorn

7. Elisa, a 14-month-old, is admitted to the hospital with laryngotracheobronchitis (croup). On assessment the nurse would expect to find:
   A. Cyanosis and dyspnea
   B. Productive coughing and a high fever
   C. Pale laryngeal tissue and dyspnea
   D. Barking cough and inspiratory stridor

8. The plan of care for a child with bronchitis should include:
   A. Ensuring bed rest and minimal oral fluid intake
   B. Keeping room air cool and dry
   C. Encouraging shallow inspiration to decrease chest pain
   D. Using expectorants and coughing to clear secretions

9. A 5-month-old child is admitted to your unit with bronchiolitis. Assessment reveals the following: temperature 102°F, apical pulse 154 bpm, respirations 68, and irritability. Oxygen therapy is ordered. The nurse understands that the rationale for this therapy is to:
   A. Liquefy secretions
   B. Promote rest
   C. Relieve hypoxemia
   D. Decrease coughing

10. When developing a teaching plan for a group of parents about cystic fibrosis, the nurse would be least likely to include which statement?
    A. It is inherited as an autosomal recessive trait.
    B. It occurs in about 1 in 2,000 births, mostly among whites.
    C. Symptoms include patchy consolidations and tumors throughout the lungs.
    D. It has an improved mortality rate, with 50% of children now living to the age of 21.

ALTERNATE FORMAT QUESTIONS

Fill in the Blank

Supply the missing term or the information requested.

1. The first indicator of airway obstruction in children is ______________________.

2. The respiratory centers are located in the ______ and the ______________________.

Multiple-Answer Multiple Choice

Circle the letter(s) corresponding to the appropriate answer(s). Select all that apply.

1. Which of the following test results aids in the diagnosis of cystic fibrosis?
   A. Decreased levels of pancreatic enzymes in duodenal secretions
   B. Elevated plasma cholesterol
   C. Elevated chloride in sweat
   D. Increased fat content of the stool
   E. Decreased chloride in sweat

2. It is very important that the nurse prevent aspiration following bronchoscopy. Which of the following interventions would be appropriate?
   A. Feed the client slowly for the first hour.
   B. Keep the client NPO until the gag reflex has returned.
   C. Provide postural drainage for the first postoperative day.
   D. Keep head elevated at 90 degrees for the first postoperative day.
   E. Maintain the bed flat and the client prone for the first hour.

CHAPTER 41

Nursing Care of the Child With a Cardiovascular Disorder

CHAPTER OVERVIEW

Chapter 41 provides an overview of various cardiovascular conditions found in children. The potential effects of these conditions on the physical and psychological growth and development of the child are discussed. The use of the nursing process to plan and provide care for the client and for the family coping with a cardiovascular disorder is explored. The case study provides the student with an exercise involving preparation and management of a client undergoing a cardiac catheterization.

LEARNING OBJECTIVES

After mastering the content in this chapter, you should be able to do the following:

1. Describe the common cardiovascular disorders of childhood.
2. Assess a child with cardiovascular dysfunction.
3. Use the nursing process to formulate and address nursing diagnoses for the child with a cardiovascular disorder.
4. Identify National Health Goals related to cardiovascular disorders and children that nurses could be instrumental in helping the nation achieve.
5. Use critical thinking to analyze ways that nursing care of children with cardiovascular disorders could be more family-centered.
6. Synthesize knowledge of cardiovascular disorders with the nursing process to achieve quality maternal and child health nursing care.

KEY TERMS

acyanotic heart disease
afterload
balloon angioplasty
cardiac catheterization
contractility
cyanosis
cyanotic heart disease
diastole
echocardiography
electrocardiogram
fluoroscopy
heart failure
hypertension
innocent heart murmur
left-to-right shunt
organic heart murmur
phonocardiography
polycythemia
postcardiac surgery syndrome
postperfusion syndrome
preload
right-to-left shunt
systole
vasculitis

■ Mastering the Information

MATCHING

Match the terms in Column I with a definition, example, or related statement from Column II. Place the letter corresponding to the answer in the space provided.

COLUMN I

1. ____Endocarditis
2. ____Dyslipidemia
3. ____Patent ductus arteriosus
4. ____Polycythemia
5. ____Postperfusion syndrome
6. ____Chest radiography
7. ____Atrial septal defect
8. ____Phonocardiography
9. ____Echocardiography
10. ____Pulmonic stenosis
11. ____Truncus arteriosus
12. ____Heart failure

13. ____Kawasaki disease
14. ____Calcium chloride
15. ____Rheumatic fever

COLUMN II

a. Agent used to increased heart contractility, possibly in place of epinephrine; contraindicated in patients with digitalis toxicity
b. An extreme increase in red blood cells in an attempt to increase tissue oxygenation
c. Fever, splenomegaly, general malaise, and a maculopapular rash that occurs after open heart surgery
d. Condition involving increased fatty acid level in the blood
e. Infection of the valves of the heart, generally caused by streptococci
f. Abnormal communication between the two atria where blood flows from left to right
g. Left-to-right shunting of blood due to connection of the pulmonary artery to the aorta
h. Autoimmune condition that typically results in a wide pulse pressure and systolic-diastolic murmur
i. Condition that involves a narrowing of the pulmonary valve
j. One major artery arises from the left and right ventricles instead of separate vessels
k. Condition resulting when the myocardium of the heart cannot circulate and pump enough blood to supply the tissues of the body
l. Mucocutaneous lymph node syndrome occurring almost exclusively in children before puberty
m. A diagram of heart sounds translated into electrical energy by a microphone placed on the child's chest
n. An ultrasound produced by high-frequency sound waves used to locate and study the movements and dimensions of cardiac structures
o. Study that furnishes an accurate picture of the heart size and contour and size of the heart chambers

SHORT ANSWER

Supply the missing term or the information requested.

1. In heart defects in which a connection exists between the right and left heart, the blood through the connective structure flows from ________ to ________.
2. Newborns and infants with heart disease are commonly brought to the health care facility by parents because the child is having ________.
3. Chest tubes inserted in a child during open heart surgery will include an upper tube draining ________ and a lower one draining ________.
4. Rejection after cardiac transplant can occur as ________, ________, or ________ forms.
5. ________ refers to a structural or functional abnormality of the ventricular myocardium that occurs after an infection and results in severe dilation of the left or both ventricles.
6. In addition to fever, three other criteria for the diagnosis of Kawasaki disease are ________, ________, and ________.
7. List the prenatal and birth information that should be discussed while obtaining a nursing history for a child with a cardiovascular disorder.
8. Relate two major areas of information to be discussed with parents taking home their child who has a heart disorder.
9. Discuss the preparatory teaching necessary for a child and family before open heart surgery.
10. Describe how innocent and organic murmurs differ relative to duration, quality, and intensity.

■ Applying Your Knowledge

CASE STUDY

Harriette Borders, age 5, has been complaining of headaches and fatigue. She also experienced syncope at school. She was seen at the pediatrician's office and referred to the children's hospital for a cardiac catheterization. Mr. and Mrs. Borders bring Harriette to the hospital and you are assigned to care for her during the procedure.

1. Mrs. Borders was instructed not to allow Harriette to eat or drink fluids after midnight the morning before the procedure. What was the reasoning for these instructions?
2. What is the purpose of the cardiac catheter?
3. Why is placement of the catheter in the vein necessary as part of the procedure?

4. What is the nursing responsibility regarding the vessel chosen for catheterization?

5. The child undergoing this procedure is awake during the process. It is likely that she would be anxious, afraid, and uncooperative if not prepared appropriately. What are some measures you can use to reduce Harriette's anxiety?

6. When Harriette returns from the procedure, what is the most important postoperative nursing diagnosis?

7. You inform Mr. Borders that Harriette must lie flat in bed for 3 hours after returning to her room. Explain the physiologic rationale for this statement.

CRITICAL INQUIRY EXERCISE

1. Prepare a plan to teach cardiopulmonary resuscitation to family members of a child with a cardiac anomaly.

2. Prepare a teaching plan to instruct the family on how exercising and modifying nutritional intake can improve cardiovascular health. Include the National Health Goals in your plan.

3. Prepare for a class presentation an outline contrasting the hemodynamics of cyanotic and acyanotic heart disease.

CRITICAL EXPLORATION

Visit a neonatal intensive care unit and assess various infants. Identify heart sounds, differences in vital signs, and feeding problems.

■ Practicing for NCLEX

MULTIPLE-CHOICE QUESTIONS

Circle the letter that corresponds to the best answer for each question.

1. A child with coarctation of the aorta might require which of the following nursing interventions?
   A. Assisting the child and parents with coping with this terminal illness
   B. Informing females with the condition that pregnancy seldom causes problems
   C. Reassuring the child and parents that post-operative abdominal pain will subside
   D. Scheduling the surgery during early infancy to prevent complications

2. Nursing care of the child with an atrial septal defect would involve which of the following?
   A. Reporting splitting of the second heart sound immediately as a serious complication
   B. Preparing the child and family for cardiac catheterization
   C. Monitoring the diastolic murmur over the apical area that is diagnostic of the condition
   D. Teaching parents about the lifelong medications required to control the condition

3. Parents of a child with a pacemaker must be taught:
   A. The procedure for cardiac defibrillation in case a dysrhythmia occurs
   B. How to take the child's pulse accurately to determine pacemaker function
   C. To change the pacemaker battery every year if symptoms indicate the need
   D. That prolonged hiccuping is a harmless side effect from pacemaker leads

4. Which of the following findings may be noted in a child with coarctation of the aorta?
   A. Low blood pressure in the upper extremities
   B. High blood pressure in the lower extremities
   C. A history of headaches and nosebleeds
   D. A capillary refill of less than 5 seconds

5. Which of the following would be most effective in reducing the workload of the heart of a child with heart failure?
   A. Bed rest in a semi-Fowler's position
   B. Digoxin administration daily, IV or orally
   C. Oxygen therapy by mask, cannula, or tent
   D. Intravenous infusion of 2,000 to 3,000 mL/day

6. Which of the following is true about congestive heart failure?
   A. Edema is an early symptom of heart failure in children.
   B. Irritability and restlessness may indicate abdominal pain from hepatomegaly.
   C. Left heart failure initially presents with jugular vein distention.
   D. Right heart failure results in pulmonary edema as an initial sign.

7. Reduction of complications from rheumatic fever can be accomplished through which of the following interventions?
   A. Administration of penicillin to children with strep throat or impetigo
   B. Beginning speech therapy to reverse damage after antibiotics are completed
   C. Pushing children with chorea to perform activities requiring fine motor movement to strengthen muscles
   D. Withholding salicylates to prevent joint hemorrhage

8. Nursing interventions for a child with Kawasaki disease may include which of the following?
   A. Maintaining heavy bed coverings and clothing to keep the child warm and comfortable
   B. Palpating skin temperature and assessing capillary filling in fingers and toes
   C. Performing range-of-motion exercises to joints hourly to prevent contractures
   D. Withholding all aspirin-containing medications to prevent platelet agglutination

9. Hypertension in children most commonly:
   A. Manifests frequent severe symptoms
   B. Cannot be treated with diet and daily exercise
   C. Results as a secondary manifestation of another disease
   D. Will resolve before adolescence without treatment if it is primary hypertension

ALTERNATE FORMAT QUESTIONS

Fill in the Blank

Supply the missing term or the information requested.

1. ______ ______ is the most frequent cause of cardiac arrest in children.

2. Identify the name of the congenital heart disorder described.
   A. Includes pulmonary artery stenosis, ventricular septal defect, dextroposition of the aorta and right ventricular hypertrophy.______________
   B. The aorta rises from the right ventricle instead of the left ventricle; usually accompanied by atrial and septal defects. ______________
   C. The tricuspid valve is closed and the foramen ovale and ductus arteriosus remain patent.

      ____

3. One of the first signs of congestive heart failure in children is ______________.

Multiple-Answer Multiple Choice

Circle the letter(s) corresponding to the appropriate answer(s). Select all that apply.

1. Select the appropriate intervention(s) for a child with a cardiovascular disorder.
   A. Ambulating a child immediately after a cardiac catheterization to prevent pulmonary atelectasis
   B. Assessing the skin surface of all black children to determine if cyanosis is present
   C. Loosening the dressing on the cardiac catheter site to promote comfort
   D. Bringing the parents of a child awaiting open heart surgery to the intensive care unit before surgery to prepare them
   E. Administering intravenous fluids liberally and rapidly to a child after open heart surgery to replace massive blood loss
   F. Reassuring the parents of a child with a ventricular septal defect that surgical repair is rarely required, even in large defects
   G. Preparing an infant who has just been diagnosed with pulmonic stenosis, as well as his parents, for immediate surgery

CHAPTER 42

Nursing Care of the Child With an Immune Disorder

CHAPTER OVERVIEW

Chapter 42 discusses the immune process as it relates to childhood illness. Immune disorders noted in childhood are reviewed. The use of the nursing process to plan and provide care for the child and the family coping with an immune disorder is explored.

LEARNING OBJECTIVES

After mastering the content in this chapter, you should be able to do the following:

1. Describe the immune process as it relates to childhood illness.
2. Assess the child with a disorder of the immune system.
3. Use the nursing process to formulate and address nursing diagnoses for the child with a disorder of the immune system.
4. Identify National Health Goals related to immune disorders and children that nurses could be instrumental in helping the nation achieve.
5. Identify areas related to care of the child with an immune disorder that could benefit from additional nursing research.
6. Use critical thinking to analyze ways that nursing care for the child with an immune disorder can be more family-centered.
7. Synthesize knowledge of immune disorders and the nursing process to achieve quality child health nursing care.

KEY TERMS

allergen
anaphylaxis
angioedema
antigen
autoimmunity
B lymphocyte
cell-mediated immunity
chemotaxis
complement
contact dermatitis
cytotoxic response
cytotoxic T cells
delayed hypersensitivity
environmental control
hapten formation
helper T cell
humoral immunity
hypersensitivity response
hyposensitization
immune response
immunity
immunocompetent cells
immunogen
killer T cell
lymphokines
lysis
macrophage
memory cell
phagocytosis
plasma cell
suppressor T cell
T lymphocyte
tolerance
urticaria

■ Mastering the Information

MATCHING

Match the terms in Column I with a definition, example, or related statement from Column II. Place the letter corresponding to the answer in the space provided.

COLUMN I

1. ____Antigen
2. ____Cell-mediated immunity
3. ____Hapten formation
4. ____Immunocompetent cells
5. ____Immunogen
6. ____Lymphokines
7. ____Memory cell
8. ____Phagocytosis
9. ____Serum sickness
10. ____Suppressor cells

COLUMN II

a. The neutralization of pathogens through ingestion by white blood cells
b. Secretion by cytotoxic cells that contain or prevent migration of antigens
c. Foreign substance capable of stimulating an immune response
d. Responsible for retaining the formula or ability to produce specific immunoglobulins
e. A hypersensitivity reaction to a foreign serum antigen or drug
f. A nonantigenic substance that becomes antigenic when combined with a higher-weight molecule
g. T cells that reduce the production of immunoglobulins against a specific antigen
h. An antigen that can be readily destroyed by an immune response
i. When antibodies are formed in response to a particular antigen; acquired through T-lymphocyte activity
j. Cells capable of resisting foreign invaders

SHORT ANSWER

Supply the missing term or the information requested.

1. Provide the type of primary immunodeficiency for each description.
   A. Cellular immune response remains adequate; child has resistance to viral, fungal, and parasitic infections, but all levels of immunoglobulins are abnormally low:

      ____

   B. Infection of surfaces exposed to the external environment and normally protected by mucus are common along with atopic diseases:

      ____

2. Human immunodeficiency virus (HIV) is spread by two primary routes in the adult population: ——— contact and ——— contact.
3. ——— results from an inability to distinguish self from nonself, causing the immune system to carry out immune responses against normal cells and tissue.
4. Assessment of the exact symptoms of an allergy is important in helping to identify the ———.
5. The three goals for therapy in childhood allergy situations are to ———, ———, and ———.
6. The best way to identify the specific allergies in a child with food allergies is the use of a ——— ——— or an elimination diet.
7. State two measures a parent can take to decrease allergies in the bedroom, in the living room, and at school.
8. Compare seborrheic dermatitis and infantile eczema in terms of the presence of itching, age of onset, length of disease, and mood of the child.
9. Differentiate between congenital and acquired immunodeficiency disorders.
10. Discuss the purpose and use of skin testing when assessing allergies in children.

■ Applying Your Knowledge

CASE STUDY

José is a 4-year-old with a primary B-cell, IgA-type immune deficiency disorder. He is admitted to your unit with an upper respiratory tract infection. His parents are concerned that his brothers and sisters will also contract the immune deficiency, so they won't let their other children play with José.

1. What is the most important concept you must include in a teaching plan for José's parents?
2. How would you approach his parents regarding their fears about José's siblings?
3. What concerns would you have about caring for José?

CRITICAL INQUIRY EXERCISE

1. Prepare a teaching plan on the diagnosis of allergic rhinitis for a child and his or her family.
2. What would your response be to a fellow nurse who refuses to care for a client with contact dermatitis because the nurse fears becoming infected?

CRITICAL EXPLORATION

During a clinical experience, monitor care provided to a client with AIDS. Note the precautions used in care and the client's emotional response to the care and care providers. Note the care that you felt was particularly good, as well as ways in which care, physical and emotional, might have been improved.

■ Practicing for NCLEX

MULTIPLE-CHOICE QUESTIONS

Circle the letter that corresponds to the best answer for each question.

1. Nurses can help the nation achieve health goals related to human immunodeficiency virus by doing which of the following?
   A. Instructing young people that IV drugs are safer than oral drugs, although both are bad
   B. Encouraging drug addicts to share needles with friends only, if they must use drugs
   C. Educating children about the importance of using condoms or practicing abstinence
   D. Avoiding discussions related to sex in adolescents younger than 18 years old

2. Janice has a deficiency that affects her humoral immunity. The nurse prepares to teach Janice about this condition as resulting from inadequate:
   A. B cells
   B. Antigens
   C. T cells
   D. Allergens

3. When teaching a group of parents about atopic disorders, which of the following would the nurse be least likely to include in the discussion?
   A. Asthma
   B. Hay fever
   C. Atopic dermatitis
   D. Serum sickness

4. Which of the following actions would be appropriate when providing care to a child with a hypersensitivity condition?
   A. Having a syringe filled with a 1:5 dilution of the antigen on hand to counteract an unexpected anaphylactic reaction from skin testing
   B. Keeping the child at the health care setting for 30 minutes after the hyposensitization process
   C. Excluding the child with allergies from planning methods of environmental control to avoid resistance to the changes
   D. Encouraging parents who know of familial allergy patterns to bottle-feed infants

ALTERNATE FORMAT QUESTIONS

Fill in the Blank

Supply the missing term or the information requested.

1. Congenital immunodeficiencies usually manifest after the first ——— months of life.

2. When a child is stung by a bee, the immediate action should be to apply ——— to the site to minimize the absorption of the venom.

Multiple-Answer Multiple Choice

Circle the letter(s) corresponding to the correct answer. Select all that apply.

1. Select the appropriate intervention(s).
   A. Anticipate treating a child who faints after an insect bite or drug injection for possible anaphylaxis.
   B. Administer a smaller-than-normal dosage of foreign serum to a child known to manifest serum sickness.
   C. Do not allow children who develop urticaria as a result of exposure to extreme temperatures to swim in cold water.
   D. Instruct parents of children with atopic dermatitis to cover the area with dressings coated in Burow's solution.
   E. Teach parents that all of the solution in an Epi-Pen must be ejected on injection.

CHAPTER 43

Nursing Care of the Child With an Infectious Disorder

CHAPTER OVERVIEW

Chapter 43 discusses common infectious disorders of childhood. The nursing techniques required to address the needs of children and their families when coping with an infectious disease are reviewed. The use of the nursing process to plan and provide care for the child with an infectious disease and his or her family is explored.

LEARNING OBJECTIVES

After mastering the content in this chapter, you should be able to do the following:

1. Describe the causes and course of common infectious disorders of childhood.
2. Assess the child with an infection.
3. Use the nursing process to identify and address nursing diagnoses related to infection in children.
4. Identify National Health Goals related to infectious disorders and children that nurses could be instrumental in helping the nation achieve.
5. Identify areas of nursing care related to children with infectious diseases that could benefit from additional nursing research.
6. Use critical thinking to analyze ways that care of the child with an infection can be more family-centered.
7. Synthesize knowledge of infectious diseases and the nursing process to achieve quality child health nursing care.

KEY TERMS

catarrhal stage
chain of infection
complement
convalescent period
enanthem
exanthem
exotoxin
fomites
incubation period
interferon
Koplik's spots
means of transmission
portal of entry
portal of exit
prodromal period
reservoir
septicemia
susceptible host
toxoid

■ Mastering the Information

MATCHING

Match the terms in Column I with a definition, example, or related statement from Column II. Place the letter corresponding to the answer in the space provided.

COLUMN I

1. ____Pathogens
2. ____Prodromal period
3. ____Chain of infection
4. ____Reservoir
5. ____Fomites
6. ____Herpes labialis
7. ____Exanthem
8. ____Illness
9. ____Interferon
10. ____Furuncle
11. ____Vector

COLUMN II

a. A rash on the skin
b. Organisms that cause disease in children
c. A time between the beginning of nonspecific symptoms and specific symptoms
d. The stage during which specific symptoms are evident
e. The method by which organisms spread and enter a new individual to cause disease
f. The container or place in which organisms grow and reproduce
g. Inanimate objects such as soil, food, or water
h. Living carriers such as insects
i. A cold sore, representing a type 1 herpesvirus invasion
j. A lymphokine; prevent cells from being host to more than one virus at a time
k. An infection of the hair follicle; a boil

SHORT ANSWER

Supply the missing term or the information requested.

1. The sources of pathogens are classified as ___________, ___________, ___________, ___________, and ___________.
2. Once the rabies disease process begins, rabies is invariably ___________.
3. The incubation period for mumps is _________ to ________ days, and the period of communicability is shortly before or after the onset of __________.
4. Discuss the method through which organisms are spread, listing the elements necessary to complete the chain of infection.
5. Discuss circumstances that cause a child to be susceptible to infection.
6. Discuss why a child should be skin tested for tuberculosis before measles vaccination.
7. Describe the universal precautions health care providers should take in all clinical settings.
8. List the signs and symptoms of scarlet fever.

■ Applying Your Knowledge

CASE STUDY

Petro Juan, age 17, is admitted to your unit with infectious mononucleosis. Petro is complaining of tiredness but his parents are encouraging him to be more active to regain his strength.

1. What are some factors that contributed to Petro being a susceptible (at-risk) host for infection?
2. What would be your response to Petro's parents regarding their approach to Petro's treatment?
3. What factors should be included in the nutritional plan of care?

CRITICAL INQUIRY EXERCISE

1. If your patient was on strict isolation and you observed another health care professional entering the patient's room without wearing protective items, what would you do?
2. A patient is admitted to your unit, and you suspect from his history that he has had a recent exposure to a person with an active case of varicella. Your hospital requires a physician's order before placing a patient on respiratory isolation. What actions would you take?

CRITICAL EXPLORATION

While on a clinical unit, provide care for a child on various types of isolation (e.g., respiratory, enteric). Compare precautions taken with each patient when emptying urine, providing the bedpan, or collecting and testing a blood specimen.

■ Practicing for NCLEX

MULTIPLE-CHOICE QUESTIONS

Circle the letter that corresponds to the best answer for each question.

1. Belinda, age 6, has been diagnosed with infectious mononucleosis. The nurse should do which of the following?
   A. Encourage Belinda to return to school and normal physical activity after 10 days.
   B. Limit Belinda's fluids to decrease the workload of the spleen.
   C. Keep Belinda in bed for a week or more with quiet games and books.
   D. Push on Belinda's upper stomach daily and report any complaints of tenderness.

2. When a child is scratched by a cat, the parents should be instructed to do which of the following?
   A. Destroy the animal to prevent subsequent attacks.
   B. Submit the animal for a blood test to diagnose cat scratch disease.
   C. Monitor the child for irritability and changes in level of consciousness.
   D. Place ice on enlarged nodes to control and decrease swelling.

3. To prevent exposure to Lyme disease, an individual should do which of the following?
   A. Wear dark-colored clothing to avoid attracting ticks.
   B. Inspect the skin of children exposed to wooded areas for tick bites.
   C. Apply calamine lotion to tick bite areas immediately to remove poison.
   D. If a tick is noted on the skin, remove it quickly using your fingernails.

ALTERNATE FORMAT QUESTIONS

Fill in the Blank

Supply the missing term or the information requested.

1. ——— is the time between the invasion of an organism and the onset of symptoms of infection.
2. ——— is a common rickettsial disease transmitted by a tick.
3. ——— enters the body through the skin, migrates to the intestinal tract, and thrives on blood, causing severe anemia.
4. ——— is a highly contagious viral infection that spreads by direct or indirect contact of saliva or vesicles, possibly being reactivated at a later time.
5. ———, caused by the papillomavirus, represents one of the most common dermatologic diseases in children.
6. A serious complication from mumps occurring in males over the age of puberty is ———.

Multiple-Answer Multiple Choice

Circle the letter(s) corresponding to the appropriate answer(s). Select all that apply.

1. Which of the following interventions are appropriate?
   A. Instruct parents to wash impetigo skin crusts daily with half-strength peroxide.
   B. Assess for hypersensitivity to iodine or shellfish before administering the antitoxin to a child with diphtheria.
   C. Explain to parents that the child with pertussis (whooping cough) must be watched closely for airway obstruction.
   D. Monitor the client suspected of exposure to tetanus for redness and pus at the site of entrance of the bacillus.
   E. Inform parents that a temperature of 101° to 102°F is an expected symptom in children with tetanus.
   F. Instruct parents to monitor children with possible tick bites for signs and symptoms of Rocky Mountain spotted fever.
   G. Teach parents of children with pet birds that if the bird doesn't appear ill, the child cannot contract psittacosis.
   H. Instruct parents of school-age children with head lice that lice infestation can occur regardless of personal hygiene.
   I. Wash the skin of a patient who has scabies with warm soapy water daily to destroy the mites.
   J. Examine a child's anal area to detect the presence of pinworms.

CHAPTER 44

Nursing Care of the Child With a Hematologic Disorder

CHAPTER OVERVIEW

The disease process of some blood disorders in children may be insidious; presenting symptoms in the early stage of the disease may not alert parents. However, many of these illnesses can become life-threatening. The nurse must be able to synthesize knowledge of findings from systems assessments with the signs and symptoms of hematologic disorders. Chapter 44 provides the student with the knowledge to care for the child and family with a hematologic disorder. The case study involves the altered hematologic processes in a sickle cell crisis.

LEARNING OBJECTIVES

After mastering the content in this chapter, you should be able to do the following:

1. Describe the major hematologic disorders of childhood, such as sickle cell anemia, iron-deficiency anemia, hemophilia, and thalassemia.
2. Assess the child with a hematologic disorder.
3. Use the nursing process to identify and address nursing diagnoses for the child with a hematologic disorder.
4. Identify National Health Goals related to children with hematologic disorders that nurses could be instrumental in helping the nation achieve.
5. Use critical thinking to analyze ways that nursing care for a child with a hematologic disorder could be more family-centered.
6. Synthesize knowledge of hematologic disorders in children with the nursing process to achieve quality child health nursing care.

KEY TERMS

agranulocytes
allogeneic transplantation
aplastic anemias
autologous transplantation
blood dyscrasias
blood plasma
direct bilirubinleukopenia
erythroblasts
erythrocytes
erythropoietin
granulocytes
Heinz bodies
hemochromatosis
hemoglobin
hemolysis
hemosiderosis
hypodermoclysis
leukocytes
sickle cell crisis
megakaryocytes
normoblasts
pancytopenia
petechiae
plethora
poikilocytic
polycythemia
priapism
purpura
reticulocytes
sickle cell trait
synergeneic transplantation
thrombocytes
thrombocytopenia

■ Mastering the Information

MATCHING

Match the terms in Column I with a definition, example, or related statement from Column II. Place the letter corresponding to the answer in the space provided.

COLUMN I

1. ____Heinz bodies
2. ____Leukopenia
3. ____Disseminated intravascular coagulation
4. ____Plethora
5. ____Allogeneic transplantation
6. ____Purpura
7. ____Normochromic anemia
8. ____Hypochromic anemia
9. ____Erythropoietin
10. ____Poikilocytic

COLUMN II

a. Acquired disorder of blood clotting that results from excessive trauma
b. Transfer of bone marrow from an immune-compatible donor via intravenous infusion to the recipient
c. Odd-shaped particles in red blood cells
d. Impaired production of erythrocytes by the bone marrow or loss of circulatory red blood cells
e. Marked reddened appearance of the skin
f. Red blood cells that are irregular in shape
g. Results from a reduced number of white blood cells
h. A hormone produced by the kidneys that stimulates the formation of red blood cells
i. Hemorrhagic rash or small hemorrhages occurring in the superficial layer of the skin
j. Inadequate hemoglobin synthesis accompanied by a reduction in the diameter of cells when hemoglobin synthesis is inadequate

SHORT ANSWER

Supply the missing term or the information requested.

1. The ultimate therapy for treating acquired aplastic anemia is ___________ ___________ ___________.
2. _______ is excessive destruction of red blood cells.
3. ________ ________ ________ ________ is a potentially lethal immunologic response of donor T cells against the tissue of the recipient.

■ Applying Your Knowledge

CASE STUDY

Phyllis, age 12, has been experiencing problems from sickle cell anemia since she was 1 year old. She has been admitted to the pediatric ward of a children's hospital with an admitting diagnosis of sickle cell crisis.

1. Since Phyllis has previously been diagnosed with sickle cell anemia, what characteristics would the physician most probably find on this admission?
2. What are the primary nursing goals when caring for Phyllis?
3. What precautionary measures are there to consider when administering IV fluids to Phyllis?
4. What findings on the assessment would suggest that Phyllis needs oxygen supplementation?

CRITICAL INQUIRY EXERCISE

1. Develop a nursing care plan that addresses the nursing process to care for the patient with aplastic anemia.
2. Create a list of foods that would be most appropriate for a school-age child with iron-deficiency anemia.

CRITICAL EXPLORATION

Attend a camp for children with sickle cell anemia. Assess the program's objectives and goals for camp participants.

■ Practicing for NCLEX

MULTIPLE-CHOICE QUESTIONS

Circle the letter that corresponds to the best answer for each question.

1. Which of the following foods is the best source of iron for the infant?
   A. Human breast milk
   B. Iron-fortified cereals
   C. Vegetables
   D. Fruit
2. Which of the following drugs is contraindicated for a child who is diagnosed as deficient in glucose 6-phosphate dehydrogenase (G-6PD)?
   A. Acetylsalicylic acid
   B. Acetaminophen
   C. Ampicillin
   D. Tetracycline

3. Mrs. Hill brings her 10-month-old son, Keith, to the emergency room with a temperature of 104.6°F. He is dehydrated and has edema of the right ankle. He is admitted to the pediatric unit. The assessment revealed a diagnosis of sickle cell crisis. The nurse explains to Mrs. Hill that Keith's signs and symptoms are a result of:
   A. Pain in the joints of the hands
   B. An amino acid deficiency
   C. An inborn error of metabolism
   D. Stasis of abnormal red blood cells in vessels

4. Which of the following might be a finding indicating sickle cell crisis in Keith?
   A. Elevated serum sodium and decreased WBCs
   B. Dry mucous membranes and priapism
   C. Loss of appetite and diarrhea
   D. Hematuria and flank pain

5. Keith's sickle cell anemia had not manifested before this age because in the first few months of his life he had:
   A. Increased protection from maternal antibodies
   B. Immature liver functioning
   C. Presence of fetal hemoglobin
   D. Increased circulatory blood volumes

ALTERNATE FORMAT QUESTIONS

Fill in the Blank

Supply the missing term or the information requested.

1. ______ are round nonnucleated bodies formed by bone marrow; normal range in count is 150,000 to 300,000/cm.

2. ______ are cells used to transport oxygen to and carry carbon dioxide away from body cells.

Multiple-Answer Multiple Choice

Circle the letter(s) corresponding to the appropriate answer(s). Select all that apply.

1. Which of the following would the nurse expect to find in a child with idiopathic thrombocytopenia?
   A. Epistaxis
   B. Asymmetrical ecchymoses on the legs
   C. Increased megakaryocytes
   D. Leukocytosis
   E. Hemolysis
   F. More than two petechiae with the tourniquet test

2. When reviewing the laboratory test results of a child diagnosed with DIC, which of the following would the nurse expect to find?
   A. Thrombocytosis
   B. Fragmented large platelets on blood smear
   C. Prolonged prothrombin time
   D. Significantly low serum fibrinogen levels
   E. Decreased fibrin split products

CHAPTER 45

Nursing Care of the Child With a Gastrointestinal Disorder

CHAPTER OVERVIEW

Chapter 45 describes the child with a disorder of the gastrointestinal system. The chapter addresses the importance of the gastrointestinal system to the entire body's ability to grow and develop in a healthy manner.

LEARNING OBJECTIVES

After mastering the content in this chapter, you should be able to do the following:

1. Describe common gastrointestinal disorders in children, such as vomiting, diarrhea, and appendicitis.
2. Assess the child with a gastrointestinal disorder.
3. Formulate nursing diagnoses for the child with a gastrointestinal disorder.
4. Develop outcomes for the child with a gastrointestinal disorder.
5. Plan nursing care with specific goals for the child with a gastrointestinal disorder
6. Implement nursing care for the child with a gastrointestinal disorder.
7. Evaluate outcomes for effectiveness and achievement of care.
8. Identify National Health Goals related to gastrointestinal disorders and children that nurses could be instrumental in helping the nation achieve.
9. Identify areas of care related to gastrointestinal disorders and children that could benefit from additional nursing research or application of evidence-based practice.
10. Analyze ways that nursing care of the child with a gastrointestinal disorder can be more family-centered.
11. Integrate knowledge of gastrointestinal disorders with the nursing process to achieve quality maternal and child health nursing care.

KEY TERMS

aganglionic megacolon
anion
appendicitis
beriberi
celiac disease
chalasia
Crohn's disease
dehydration
gastroesophageal reflux
hepatitis
hiatal hernia
inguinal hernia
insensible loss
intussusception
irritable bowel syndrome
isotonic dehydration
keratomalacia
kwashiorkor
liver transplantation
McBurney's point
Meckel's diverticulum
metabolic acidosis
necrotizing enterocolitis
nutritional marasmus
overhydration
pellagra
peptic ulcer
pyloric stenosis
rickets
steatorrhea
ulcerative colitis
volvulus
xerophthalmia

■ Mastering the Information

MATCHING

Match the terms in Column I with a definition, example, or related statement from Column II. Place the letter corresponding to the answer in the space provided.

COLUMN I

1. _____Achalasia
2. _____Aganglionic megacolon
3. _____Hiatal hernia
4. _____Isotonic dehydration
5. _____Kwashiorkor
6. _____Marasmus
7. _____Celiac disease
8. _____Hypertonic dehydration

COLUMN II

a. Loss of body water and salt in proportion to each other
b. Hirschsprung's disease, the absence of nerve cells and peristaltic waves in a section of the bowel
c. Gastroesophageal reflux due to a neuromuscular disturbance that causes a lax cardiac sphincter and lower esophagus
d. A disease caused by protein deficiency seen more frequently in children ages 1 to 3 years
e. A disease caused by deficiency of all food groups
f. Loss of body water out of proportion to salt
g. Intermittent protrusion of the stomach through the esophageal opening in the diaphragm
h. Sensitivity or abnormal immunologic response to protein, usually the gluten factor

SHORT ANSWER

Supply the missing term or the information requested.

1. The nurse is counseling Mrs. Anderson about her 8-month-old daughter, Adrienne, who has been "spitting up" food after her feedings. The problem started about 3 weeks ago. The physician tells the nurse that Adrienne has achalasia, which is also commonly called ____________ ____________.
2. The "spitting up" associated with achalasia is described as ____________ and ____________.
3. Achalasia is usually self-limiting as the esophageal sphincter matures. However, if not treated, more serious problems might develop, such as ________________ or ________________.
4. Some good advice for Mrs. Anderson would be that she use a ____________________ formula.

■ Applying Your Knowledge

CASE STUDY

Aaron is 8 months old. His birth was uneventful and he has exhibited no previous health problems. Today his mother brings him to the emergency room exhibiting symptoms of dehydration.

1. What should be the normal fluid intake and output for Aaron?
2. What are the major sources and minor sources of fluid loss for infants?
3. What are the major history and physical assessments you would make for Aaron?

CRITICAL INQUIRY EXERCISE

1. Create a teaching plan for the parents of a child with pyloric stenosis. Include preparation for hospitalization, surgery, and the recovery period.
2. Describe a process for determining if a patient's dehydration is isotonic, hypotonic, or hypertonic.

CRITICAL EXPLORATION

Visit a day-care center. Ask what the rules are regarding care of the child with diarrhea, fever, or vomiting. Observe the staff as they implement the infection control guidelines, and determine if these techniques are sufficient.

■ Practicing for NCLEX

MULTIPLE-CHOICE QUESTIONS

Circle the letter that corresponds to the best answer for each question.

1. A mother brings her 12-year-old daughter to the clinic for evaluation of complaints of a gnawing epigastric pain before meals. When questioned further, the child reports that the pain subsides after eating and she has had some episodes of vomiting. Examination reveals epigastric tenderness. The nurse interprets these findings as suggesting which of the following?
   A. Peptic ulcer disease
   B. Inflammatory bowel disease
   C. Hepatitis
   D. Pyloric stenosis

2. Which of the following laboratory results would lead the nurse to suspect a child is experiencing liver problems?
   A. Bile pigments present in stool specimen
   B. Decreased serum albumin levels
   C. Total serum bilirubin level of 1.5 mg/100 mL
   D. Urine negative for bilirubin

3. Which of the following nursing interventions might allay any guilt felt by the parents of a child with achalasia?
   A. Suggest the parents step outside the room while you feed the child so they do not view the "spitting up."
   B. Offer suggestions in positioning, since success through this measure builds confidence.
   C. Tell the parents that they were preparing the formula wrong and that this caused the condition.
   D. Reassure parents that this condition is usually due to dysentery and is not their fault.

ALTERNATE FORMAT QUESTIONS

Fill in the Blank

Supply the missing term or the information requested.

1. Metabolic _____________is indicated when the arterial blood pH is less than 7.35 and HCO_3 is below 22 mEq/L.

2. A patient who is dehydrated with an arterial blood pH :7.45 and a bicarbonate level greater than 28 mEq/L is experiencing metabolic ___________.

Multiple-Answer Multiple Choice

Circle the letter(s) corresponding to the appropriate answer(s). Select all that apply.

1. Warren is a 6-month-old infant presenting in the ED with poor intake over the past 3 days and severe diarrhea. Which of the following would the nurse expect to assess?
   A. Rapid respirations
   B. Bulging fontanel
   C. Dependent edema
   D. Dry mucous membranes
   E. Rapid thready pulse
   F. Poor skin turgor

2. Which of the following are glands that secrete saliva?
   A. Parotid
   B. Apocrine
   C. Pituitary
   D. Sublingual
   E. Submandibular

CHAPTER 46

Nursing Care of the Child With a Renal or Urinary Tract Disorder

CHAPTER OVERVIEW

Chapter 46 discusses common renal and urinary tract disorders that occur in children and the nursing care needed for these children and their families. The normal function of the renal system is reviewed. The use of the nursing process to plan and provide care for the child and family with a renal or urinary tract disorder is explored.

LEARNING OBJECTIVES

After mastering the content in this chapter, you should be able to do the following:

1. Describe common renal and urinary disorders that occur in children, such as urinary tract infection (UTI), nephrosis, and glomerulonephritis.
2. Assess a child for a renal or urinary tract disorder.
3. Use the nursing process to identify and address nursing diagnoses related to renal or urinary disorders.
4. Identify National Health Goals related to renal or urinary tract disorders and children that nurses can be instrumental in helping the nation achieve.
5. Use critical thinking to analyze methods for making nursing care of the child with a renal or urinary disorder more family-centered.
6. Synthesize knowledge of renal and urinary tract disorders with the nursing process to achieve quality child health nursing care.

KEY TERMS

acute transplant rejection
Alport's syndrome
azotemia
Bowman's capsule
dialysis
enuresis
epispadias
exstrophy of the bladder
glomerular filtration rate
glomerulonephritis
hydronephrosis
hypospadias
nephrosis
patent urachus
polycystic kidney
postural proteinuria
prune belly syndrome
vesicoureteral reflux

■ Mastering the Information

MATCHING

Match the terms in Column I with a definition, example, or related statement from Column II. Place the letter corresponding to the answer in the space provided.

COLUMN I

1. ____Prune belly syndrome
2. ____Azotemia
3. ____Cystoscopy
4. ____Cryptorchidism
5. ____Enuresis
6. ____Hypospadias
7. ____Dialysis
8. ____Acute transplant rejection
9. ____Alport's syndrome
10. ____Patent urachus

COLUMN II

a. An autosomal dominant inherited disorder with chronic renal failure
b. A fistula between the bladder and the umbilicus
c. The opening of the urethra onto the ventral or lower surface of the penis
d. Direct viewing of the bladder or ureter openings for examination
e. Undescended testes often noted with hypospadias
f. Involuntary voiding past the age when a child is expected to have attained bladder control
g. Condition manifested by fever, proteinuria, oliguria, weight gain, and hypertension developing within 3 months following transplant
h. Urethral obstruction in utero from abnormal urethral valves
i. Separation and removal of solutes from body fluid by diffusion through a semipermeable membrane
j. The accumulation of nitrogen waste in the bloodstream, often due to oliguria

SHORT ANSWER

Supply the missing term or the information requested.

1. Glomerulonephritis involves the obstruction of the glomeruli due to complement fixation activated by an ______-______ reaction, stimulated most often by a streptococcal infection.
2. The four characteristic symptoms of nephrotic syndrome are ______, ______, ______, and ______________________.
3. Children with hemolytic-uremic syndrome usually have ______ skin coloring as well as the major symptoms of ______ with proteinuria, ______, and urinary casts in urine.
4. Explain why girls are at higher risk for urinary tract infections than boys.
5. Differentiate between primary and secondary enuresis, and provide one possible physiologic and one psychological cause for secondary enuresis.
6. Compare and contrast the symptoms and treatment for nephrotic syndrome and acute glomerulonephritis.
7. Discuss the primary difference in the etiology of acute and chronic renal failure.
8. Discuss the dietary restriction of salt in a child with chronic renal failure.

■ Applying Your Knowledge

CASE STUDY

Rebecca, age 2, is admitted to your unit with dehydration and acute strep throat. After 3 days of treatment and IV fluids, you notice that Rebecca's urine output has remained low and her blood levels of nitrogen and creatinine are elevated.

1. What type of renal failure has Rebecca probably developed? What other symptoms of renal failure might you notice?
2. How would you explain Rebecca's renal condition to her parents?
3. What activity level would you expect to be ordered for Rebecca, and how would you help her maintain it?

CRITICAL INQUIRY EXERCISE

1. Prepare a teaching plan for a child discharged on continuous ambulatory peritoneal dialysis.
2. Your patient, admitted after an automobile accident, has just been diagnosed as being brain dead. What would your response be if the doctor asked you to approach the family regarding donating the patient's kidneys? When and how would you choose to approach the family?

CRITICAL EXPLORATION

Visit a dialysis unit; review three or four charts and note the various causes of renal failure.

■ Practicing for NCLEX

MULTIPLE-CHOICE QUESTIONS

Circle the letter that corresponds to the best answer for each question.

1. Which of the following interventions might be most effective in preventing glomerulonephritis?
   A. Daily administration of children's multivitamins and iron
   B. An increase in all children's fluid intake to 3 liters daily
   C. Prompt evaluation of childhood complaints of sore throat
   D. Teaching children to void promptly when the urge is felt

2. Which of the following would the nurse expect to assess in a child with acute glomerulonephritis?
   A. Blood pressure of 90/40
   B. Hypovolemia and signs of dehydration
   C. Hematuria and pulmonary edema
   D. Severe, foul-smelling diarrhea

3. The nurse could implement which of the following measures for a child who demonstrated enuresis with no apparent organic cause?
   A. Encourage the child to discuss concerns relative to changes in his environment or life.
   B. Instruct the parents never to let the child drink after dinner.
   C. Limit the fluids of children with sickle cell anemia since they are most prone to this condition.
   D. Teach parents to strictly enforce bladder training with the child.

4. Bobby, age 10, has a diagnosis of acute nephrotic syndrome. Which of the following nursing interventions would be most appropriate?
   A. Administering liberal IV and oral fluids to offset the accompanying dehydration
   B. Discussing the cushingoid effects of prescribed steroid therapy with the child and parents
   C. Reassuring the child and parents that diuretics will quickly reduce the edema
   D. Preparing the child and parents for the frequently terminal outcome of the disease

5. Which of the following would be an appropriate explanation to provide to the parents of a child with severe hypertension awaiting a renal transplant?
   A. After the child's nonfunctioning kidneys are removed, the child will have no food restrictions.
   B. Removal of only one kidney is necessary to provide room for the new kidney.
   C. Reluctant younger siblings can still serve as a kidney donor as long as the parent signs both surgery consent forms.
   D. The transplanted kidney will be placed in the abdomen, not in the usual kidney space.

ALTERNATE FORMAT QUESTIONS

Fill in the Blank

Supply the missing term or the information requested.

1. A ——— kidney is a condition involving abnormal development of the collecting tubules in which fluid-filled cysts, instead of kidney tissue, form in utero; it may be unilateral or bilateral.

2. An increase in blood levels of the products of cell metabolism such as ——— may indicate poor kidney function.

3. ——— refers to a retrograde flow of urine from the bladder into the ureters that may lead to a urinary tract infection.

Multiple-Answer Multiple Choice

Circle the letter(s) corresponding to the appropriate answer(s). Select all that apply.

1. De'Anya is a nursing student preparing a clinical care plan for her next day of practice in the hospital. She has been assigned several patients hospitalized with altered functioning of the urinary system. Which of the following would be appropriate to include in De'Anya's plan of care for her patients?
   A. Instruct the parent of the child with exstrophy of the bladder to give the infant a tub bath daily to remove sediment and maintain good hygiene.
   B. Stress the importance of repairing hypospadias before the child's maturity to prevent fertility problems.
   C. Prepare the parent of the infant with urinary tract infections for diagnostic procedures to rule out urethral stenosis or bladder reflux.
   D. Teach girls to wipe from back to front after voiding or stooling.
   E. Encourage a child with a urinary tract infection to drink liberal amounts of fluids.

2. When caring for the patient with chronic renal failure undergoing hemodialysis, which of the following would be appropriate?
   A. Instruct the parents of the child with chronic renal failure how to prepare a diet low in protein and phosphorus.
   B. Administer aluminum hydroxide, alternating with milk, to prevent ulcer formation.
   C. Encourage the child receiving corticosteroids to discuss angry feelings regarding his or her change in appearance.
   D. Monitor the child frequently during hemodialysis to detect changes in cerebral tissue perfusion.
   E. Encourage the parents to seek out time for themselves and voice frustrations and fears.

CHAPTER 47

Nursing Care of the Child With a Reproductive Disorder

CHAPTER OVERVIEW

Reproductive disorders in children range from mild infection to serious anatomic malformations. All require prompt treatment to prevent later disruption in sexual or reproductive health. Sensitive and careful questioning when assessing children with reproductive system dysfunction is essential. This chapter addresses the illnesses affecting external reproductive structures and reproductive organs. The case study affords the student the opportunity to plan the nursing care for an adolescent with an altered assessment of the male reproductive system.

LEARNING OBJECTIVES

After mastering the content in this chapter, you should be able to do the following:

1. Describe common reproductive disorders in children.
2. Assess the child with a reproductive disorder.
3. Use the nursing process to identify and address nursing diagnoses related to a child's reproductive illness.
4. Identify National Health Goals related to reproductive disorders and children that nurses can be instrumental in helping the nation achieve.
5. Identify areas related to care of children with reproductive disorders that could benefit from additional nursing research.
6. Use critical thinking to analyze ways that nursing care for the child with a reproductive disorder can be more family-centered.
7. Synthesize knowledge of reproductive disorders in children with the nursing process to achieve quality child health nursing care.

KEY TERMS

adenocarcinoma
adenosis
amenorrhea
anovulatory
colposcopy
cryptorchidism
dysmenorrhea
endometriosis
fibrocystic breast disease
gynecomastia
hermaphrodite
hydrocele
menorrhagia
metrorrhagia
mittelschmerz
orchiectomy
orchiopexy
pelvic inflammatory disease
premenstrual syndrome (PMS)
pseudohermaphrodite
sexually transmitted disease (STD)
toxic shock syndrome
varicocele
vulvovaginitis

■ Mastering the Information

MATCHING

Match the terms in Column I with a definition, example, or related statement from Column II. Place the letter corresponding to the answer in the space provided.

COLUMN I

1. ____Adenosis
2. ____Amenorrhea
3. ____Anovulatory
4. ____Hydrocele
5. ____Metrorrhagia
6. ____Orchiectomy
7. ____Pseudohermaphrodite
8. ____Toxic shock syndrome
9. ____Imperforate hymen
10. ____Pelvic inflammatory disease
11. ____Menorrhagia

COLUMN II

a. An abnormally heavy menstrual flow
b. Removal of the testes
c. Menstrual cycles that occur without the release of an egg
d. Infant with some external features of both sexes, although only ovaries or testes are present
e. Condition most frequently caused by gonorrheal infections or chlamydia
f. The formation of vaginal cysts
g. An infection caused by toxin-producing strains of staphylococcus
h. Fluid collection in the space called the processus vaginalis
i. A membranous ring of tissue totally occluding the vagina
j. Absence of menstrual flow; may suggest pregnancy
k. Bleeding between menstrual periods

SHORT ANSWER

Supply the missing term or the information requested.

1. A ——— is abnormal dilation of the veins of the spermatic cord.
2. ——— is an enlargement of the male breast.
3. ——— is failure of both testes to descend from the abdominal cavity to the scrotum.

■ Applying Your Knowledge

CASE STUDY

Peter, age 14, is seen in your clinic. He states he had sex with a girl who recently told him she was diagnosed with syphilis. He insists that nobody else know about his visit to the clinic since he can pay for the medicine himself.

1. What symptoms would you question Peter about, and what diagnostic procedures would you prepare him for?
2. What information would you include in your teaching plan for Peter?
3. What obligations would you, as a health care provider, have to keep Peter's condition strictly confidential?

CRITICAL INQUIRY EXERCISE

1. Create a poster board illustrating the female and male reproductive systems. Indicate the reproductive disorders common to both sexes and those specific to one gender or the other.
2. Write a teaching plan addressing the learning needs of a 13-year-old who indicates a desire to become sexually active. What difference, if any, would the gender of the adolescent make in the plan?

CRITICAL EXPLORATION

Arrange with your instructor to visit a health clinic that provides health care for adolescents who are sexually active. Note the health problems presented by the clients and identify the preventive measures provided by the professionals as they teach and counsel these clients.

■ Preparing for NCLEX

MULTIPLE-CHOICE QUESTIONS

Circle the letter that corresponds to the best answer for each question.

1. Baby J, 1 day old, is born with ambiguous genitalia. The nurse would incorporate teaching to help the parents as their child undergoes which of the following tests to determine gender?
   A. Blood cultures
   B. Colposcopy
   C. Karyotyping
   D. Sedimentation rate
2. A young female who has trichomoniasis may exhibit which of the following?
   A. Greenish vaginal discharge
   B. Cream cheese-like vaginal discharge
   C. Patchy white lesions on vaginal wall
   D. Frothy white or grayish-green vaginal discharge

3. Which of the following would the nurse interpret as a symptom of the final stage of syphilis?
   A. Blindness
   B. Chancre
   C. Low-grade fever
   D. Lymphadenopathy

4. After teaching an adolescent with fibrocystic breast disease about measures to reduce discomfort, the nurse determines that the client needs additional teaching when she states that which of the following would be a helpful measure?
   A. Acetaminophen
   B. Oral contraceptives
   C. Caffeine
   D. Danocrine

5. When talking to a group of adolescents about toxic shock syndrome, the nurse would include damage to which of the following as the most common method by which the organisms enter the body?
   A. Deep buccal tissue
   B. Vaginal wall tissue
   C. Urethral meatus
   D. Nasal mucous membranes

ALTERNATE FORMAT QUESTIONS

Fill in the Blank

Supply the missing term or the information requested.

1. Testicular cancer has symptoms of heaviness of the ________. It is ________ and ________ rapidly.
2. ______ is defined as experiencing abdominal pain during ovulation. The discomfort is felt on either side of the ________________, near an ovary.
3. ________ is an inflammation of the glands and prepuce of the penis.

Multiple-Answer Multiple Choice

Circle the letter(s) corresponding to the appropriate answer(s). Select all that apply.

1. When preparing a teaching plan for a group of adolescents about pelvic inflammatory disease, the nurse would include which anatomical structures as being involved?
   A. Fallopian tubes
   B. Vagina
   C. Uterus
   D. Ovaries
   E. Ovarian support structures

2. Which of the following are possible theories about the cause of premenstrual dysphoric disorder?
   A. Drop in progesterone
   B. Vitamin B complex deficiency
   C. Decreased ovarian blood supply
   D. Hyperglycemia
   E. Low calcium levels

CHAPTER 48

Nursing Care of the Child With an Endocrine or Metabolic Disorder

CHAPTER OVERVIEW

Chapter 48 reviews the care of the child with an endocrine or metabolic disorder. The chapter addresses the function of each hormone, the result of altered endocrine function, and a plan for nursing intervention. The case study helps the student understand the principles of assessing a child with an endocrine disorder.

LEARNING OBJECTIVES

After mastering the content in this chapter, you should be able to do the following:

1. Describe the structure and function of the different endocrine glands.
2. Assess a child with a disorder of endocrine function.
3. Formulate nursing diagnoses for a child with altered endocrine or metabolic function.
4. Develop appropriate outcomes for the child with endocrine or metabolic dysfunction.
5. Plan nursing care—for example, health teaching—for the child with altered endocrine or metabolic function.
6. Implement nursing care—for example, teaching insulin administration—for the child with an endocrine or metabolic disorder.
7. Evaluate outcomes to be certain that goals of nursing care were achieved.
8. Identify National Health Goals related to childhood endocrine or metabolic disorders that nurses could be instrumental in helping the nation achieve.
9. Identify areas related to care of children with endocrine or metabolic disorders that could benefit from additional nursing research or application of evidence-based practice.
10. Analyze ways that care of the child with altered endocrine or metabolic function can be family-centered.
11. Synthesize knowledge of endocrine and metabolic dysfunctions and the nursing process to ensure quality maternal and child health nursing care.

KEY TERMS

carpal spasm
exophthalmos
glycosuria
hormones
hyperfunction
hyperglycemia
hypofunction
hypoglycemia
hypothalamus
ketoacidosis
latent tetany
manifest tetany
pedal spasm
polydipsia
polyuria
sella turcica
Somogyi phenomenon

■ Mastering the Information

MATCHING

Match the terms in Column I with a definition, example, or related statement from Column II. Place the letter corresponding to the answer in the space provided.

COLUMN I

1. _____Cushing's syndrome
2. _____Latent tetany
3. _____Polydipsia
4. _____Galactosemia
5. _____Thyrotoxicosis
6. _____Kussmaul breathing
7. _____PKU
8. _____Aldosterone

 Study Guide to Accompany Maternal and Child Health Nursing: Care of the Childbearing and Childrearing Family, revised reprint, fifth edition by Joyce Young Johnson and Edna Boyd-Davis.

COLUMN II

a. Excessive thirst
b. Body's response to excessive production of thyroid hormone
c. Substance secreted in response to renin-angiotensin
d. Overproduction of the adrenal hormone cortisol
e. Deep and rapid respirations
f. Neuromuscular irritability
g. Metabolic disease inherited as an autosomal recessive trait
h. Disorder of carbohydrate metabolism

SHORT ANSWER

Supply the missing term or the information requested.

1. Type 1 (insulin-dependent) diabetes is characterized by almost no ——— secretion. The lack of insulin secretion contributes to a buildup of ——— in the bloodstream. If exogenous insulin is not administered, this person will develop ——————— and ———————.
2. Humulin-R insulin begins to work approximately ——— minutes after administration.
3. What is the primary function of the endocrine system?
4. For each hormone listed, identify the gland which secretes it.

   A. Thyroxine ____________________

   B. Somatotropin ____________________

   C. Insulin ____________________

   D. Antidiuretic hormone ____________________

   E. Aldosterone ____________________

   F. Corticotropin ____________________

■ Applying Your Knowledge

CASE STUDY

Ashley, age 5, is admitted to the children's hospital after her mother reports to the pediatrician that she has been urinating very frequently and has lost weight. Her mother also reports that she had several incidents of incontinence while playing on the playground. A careful history taken by the nurse revealed that Ashley's appetite had also increased. On admission to the hospital, laboratory studies were ordered. The results revealed a blood glucose level of 400 mg/dL.

1. The glucose tolerance test is ordered intravenously rather than orally. Why would the physician prefer this method?
2. What comfort measures should the nurse offer the child who is undergoing a fasting tolerance test?
3. What measures can be taken to lessen the discomfort for the diabetic child when frequent blood samples are needed?

CRITICAL INQUIRY EXERCISE

1. Create a blood glucose monitoring flow sheet. Be sure to include the date, blood glucose before each meal and bedtime, insulin dosage (both regular and NPH taken daily), and an explanation column where the patient can identify the reason for fluctuation in blood glucose.
2. Role-play what it is like to check your blood glucose four times a day and record the amounts on your monitoring sheet. On the next day change the numbers to indicate hyperglycemia all day. Indicate what may have contributed to the problem.

CRITICAL EXPLORATION

1. Attend a diabetes camp and offer to be a counselor in one of the cabins. Be sure to tell the camp director that diabetes is new to you and that you will need guidance.
2. Attend a meeting of the American Association of Diabetes Educators. Ask one of the certified diabetes educators about his or her job. How was certification obtained?

3. Visit a diabetes education program that has been nationally recognized by the American Diabetes Association Advisory Council. Observe patient instructions and follow-up visits.

■ Practicing for NCLEX

MULTIPLE-CHOICE QUESTIONS

Circle the letter that corresponds to the best answer for each question.

The nurse is counseling 10-year-old Shajuan and her parents about the action of insulin and its effect on blood glucose levels before meals and at bedtime. The child has been instructed to take a split dose of regular and NPH insulin twice a day. The goal is to keep all glucose levels between 80 and 150 mg/dL before meals. Shajuan has been instructed by the physician to change the insulin using pattern control.

1. The nurse explains the purpose of insulin, stating that it causes the blood glucose to:
   A. Increase
   B. Decrease
   C. Remain the same throughout
   D. Increase, then decrease

2. The nurse checks Shajuan's glucose level before bedtime and finds it to be 50 mg/dL, would be considered too low. The nurse would assess Shajuan for which of the following?
   A. Thirst
   B. Flushing
   C. Dehydration
   D. Sweating

3. Shajuan is to begin using an insulin pump. The nurse instructs her parent to test her for hypoglycemia at 2 a.m. based on the understanding that a drop in blood glucose at this time may be related to too little:
   A. Food
   B. Exercise
   C. Fluid
   D. Sodium

4. Shajuan has experienced Somogyi phenomenon. The physician is notified. Which of the following would the nurse expect the physician to order?
   A. Increase the regular insulin.
   B. Decrease the regular insulin.
   C. Increase the intake of protein at supper.
   D. Decrease the intake of protein at supper.

5. Shajuan is planning to play soccer at 3 p.m. It would be best to:
   A. Take no insulin that morning
   B. Decrease regular insulin dosage in the morning
   C. Decrease the NPH insulin dosage in the morning
   D. Increase the NPH insulin dosage in the morning

6. After teaching Shajuan and her parents about causes of hypoglycemia, the nurse determines that the teaching was effective when they state which of the following as a cause?
   A. Missing an insulin injection
   B. Missing a meal or a snack
   C. Too small an insulin dosage
   D. Too large a meal or snack

ALTERNATE FORMAT QUESTIONS

Fill in the Blank

Supply the missing term or the information requested.

1. The peak action of Humulin R insulin is within ——— to ——— hours after administration.
2. Humulin N (NPH) insulin begins to work within ——————— hours after administration.
3. Humulin N (NPH) insulin peaks within ——— to ——————— hours after administration.

Multiple-Answer Multiple Choice

Circle the letter(s) corresponding to the appropriate answer(s). Select all that apply.

1. Which of the following are correct?
   A. Growth hormone deficiency is a pituitary disorder.
   B. Hashimoto's disease interferes with thyroid gland function.
   C. Cushing syndrome is an underproduction of cortisol by the adrenal gland.
   D. The most frequently occurring pancreatic disorder in children is type 2 diabetes.
   E. Dysfunction of the parathyroid gland can cause calcium imbalances.

2. Diabetes insipidus is a disease that involves which of the following?
   A. Excessive release of the antidiuretic hormone (ADH)
   B. Trauma to the pituitary glans as a possible cause
   C. Polydipsia
   D. High urine specific gravity (1.001 to 1.005)
   E. Polyuria

CHAPTER 49

Nursing Care of the Child With a Neurologic Disorder

CHAPTER OVERVIEW

Chapter 49 discusses the care of the child with a neurologic disorder. The physiologic and psychological impact of common neurologic conditions on children at various stages of growth and development is discussed. The use of the nursing process to plan and provide care for the child with a neurologic disorder and his or her family is explored. The case study explores the nursing care of the child with a potentially life-threatening infection.

LEARNING OBJECTIVES

After mastering the content in this chapter, you should be able to do the following:

1. Describe common neurologic disorders in children.
2. Assess a child with a neurologic disorder.
3. Identify and address nursing diagnoses for the child with a neurologic disorder.
4. Identify National Health Goals for children who have neurologic disorders and elaborate on how nurses can help the identified population to achieve those goals.
5. Use critical thinking to analyze ways that care of the child with a neurologic disorder can be optimally family-centered.
6. Synthesize knowledge of neurologic disorders and the nursing process to achieve quality child health nursing care.

KEY TERMS

astereognosis
automatism
autonomic dysreflexia
autonomic nervous system (ANS)
central nervous system (CNS)
cerebrospinal fluid (CSF)
choreoathetosis
choreoid
decerebrate posturing
decorticate posturing
diplegia
doll's eye reflex
dyskinetic
dystonic
graphesthesia
hemiplegia
kinesthesia
neuron
paraplegia
peripheral nervous system (PNS)
pulse pressure
quadriplegia
status epilepticus
stereognosis

■ Mastering the Information

MATCHING

Match the terms in Column I with a definition, example, or related statement from Column II. Place the letter corresponding to the answer in the space provided.

COLUMN I

1. ____Electroencephalogram
2. ____Graphesthesia
3. ____Kinesthesia
4. ____Ataxic
5. ____Neurofibromatosis
6. ____Diplegia
7. ____Stereognosis
8. ____Decorticate posture
9. ____Decerebrate posture
10. ____Myelography

COLUMN II

a. Awkward wide-based gait
b. Subcutaneous tumors along nerve pathways, with excessive skin pigmentation and possible optic or acoustic nerve degeneration
c. The ability to recognize a shape that has been traced on the skin
d. Depiction of electrical patterns of the brain
e. The ability to distinguish movement
f. Child's arms are abducted and flexed on the chest with wrists flexed
g. Spastic cerebral palsy involvement affecting primarily the lower extremities
h. The ability to recognize an object by touch
i. Indication of nonfunctional midbrain with rigid extension and adduction of arms and wrist pronation
j. Radiographic study of spinal cord involving the use of a contrast medium

SHORT ANSWER

Supply the missing term or the information requested.

1. The nervous system consists of two separate systems, the ——— and the ——— nervous systems.
2. Tests for cerebellar function involve testing for normal ——— and ———.
3. The rate at which symptoms of intracranial pressure develop depends on the ——— and on whether the child's skull can ——— to accommodate the pressure.
4. Signs of ———, in which a child is unsure of time and place, may be the first indication of increased intracranial pressure.
5. Cerebral perfusion pressure is calculated by subtracting the mean intracranial pressure from the mean ——— pressure.
6. The major cause of meningitis in newborns is the group B hemolytic ——— organism.
7. The treatment for infant botulism consists of ——— ———.
8. Convulsions associated with high fever are most common in ——— ——— aged children.

■ Applying Your Knowledge

CASE STUDY

Mrs. Vereen has brought Shawn to the emergency room with an elevated temperature. Shawn is 4 years old and has had a cold for several days. Shawn's temperature on assessment was 104°F orally. He began to have a seizure during admission and was immediately taken to the treatment room. After some initial testing, he was diagnosed with *H. influenzae* meningitis.

1. How was the diagnosis confirmed?
2. Why should the nurse assess Shawn's skin for changes during assessments?
3. How is this disease treated? What is the impending complication if left untreated?
4. Should there be a concern for siblings and family members of the child with bacterial meningitis?

CRITICAL INQUIRY EXERCISE

1. Develop an abbreviated assessment that a soccer coach could use to assess an injured child with a mobility problem. Include advice the coach must give to the persons who may want to assist him or her before professional help arrives.
2. Prepare a teaching plan stressing the importance of health care to prevent accidents; customize this plan to teach a parent group in a day-care setting. Include the National Health Goals as they relate to upper respiratory infections, the relationship of a disease and age frequency, and bike riding on streets.

CRITICAL EXPLORATION

1. While on a pediatric clinical unit, perform a neurologic assessment on a client with no known neurologic conditions and on a client with a neurologic condition affecting neuromuscular or cerebral function. Note the differences in findings.

2. Observe the room of a client who has a history of seizures, or areas in which precautions should be taken, and note the seizure precautions taken for that client's safety.

■ Practicing for NCLEX

MULTIPLE-CHOICE QUESTIONS

Circle the letter that corresponds to the best answer for each question.

1. Melle, age 7, is admitted to your unit after an automobile accident. You would suspect increased intracranial pressure if your assessment revealed which of the following?
   A. Bradycardia
   B. Decreased pulse pressure
   C. Hypotensive blood pressure
   D. Tachypnea

2. A doll's eye reflex:
   A. Can be used to assess a comatose child neurologically
   B. Indicates increased intracranial pressure
   C. Results when a child turns his or her eyes to the left as his or her head is turned to the left rapidly
   D. Represents an abnormal neurologic finding

3. Billy, age 2, has been diagnosed with cerebral palsy. The nurse should explain which of the following to Billy's parents?
   A. Cerebral palsy involves a progressive nerve degeneration.
   B. Contractures are unavoidable since ambulation is impossible.
   C. The brain damage that occurred at birth can be repaired with surgery when the child is older.
   D. Two children with cerebral palsy may exhibit totally different symptoms and abilities.

4. A child with Guillain-Barré syndrome will require which of the following nursing interventions?
   A. Oral feeding to maintain the muscles of mastication
   B. Explaining to parents that steroids will be effective in halting the paralysis
   C. Immobilizing extremities to decrease stimulation of muscle spasm
   D. Inserting an indwelling catheter into the bladder to monitor urine output

5. To decrease the incidence of spinal cord injury in children and adolescents, the nurse should do which of the following?
   A. Caution children and adolescents against diving into shallow water.
   B. Encourage the intake of vitamins A and C to minimize spinal cord injury.
   C. Instruct adolescents to ride motorcycles instead of driving cars.
   D. Teach back exercises to children to strengthen their weak vertebrae.

6. A child with a cervical spinal injury should be watched very carefully for which of the following?
   A. Diarrhea and hypoactive bowel sounds during the second recovery phase
   B. Hyperreflexia of the bladder during the first recovery phase
   C. Profuse diaphoresis during the second recovery phase
   D. Respiratory distress during the first recovery phase

7. Which of the following would lead the nurse to suspect that a child with a spinal cord injury is developing autonomic dysreflexia?
   A. Bradycardia and flushed face
   B. Headache and hypertension
   C. Hypertension and pallor
   D. Pale skin and dizziness

8. Which of the following is true about the third phase of spinal cord recovery?
   A. Autonomic dysreflexia is a common occurrence.
   B. Spasticity of muscles and reflexes is noted.
   C. Flaccid paralysis of the diaphragm and skeletal muscles is present.
   D. Permanent limitation of motor and sensory function can be assessed.

9. Benje, age 7, is admitted to the emergency room with suspected spinal cord injury after an automobile accident. Which of the following nursing interventions would be appropriate?
   A. Move the child from the admission stretcher to a firm examining table on admission.
   B. Hyperextend the head if respiratory resuscitation is necessary.
   C. Remove any hard head coverings and replace with a support neck brace.
   D. Maintain spinal immobilization during neurologic assessments.

10. Nursing care of the child who has suffered a spinal cord injury may include which of the following interventions?
   A. Pushing carbonated beverages during the first phase of recovery to acidify urine
   B. Using Credé's maneuver to establish a defecation pattern
   C. Helping the child and family adjust to permanent mobility loss during the first recovery phase
   D. Supporting the child and family during the grieving process after the second recovery phase

ALTERNATE FORMAT QUESTIONS

Fill in th

Circle the letter that corresponds to the best answer for each question.

1. Indicate if the following actions test sensory, motor, or cerebellar function.

a. Asking a child to touch each finger on one hand with the thumb of that hand in rapid succession

____

b. Asking a child to resist your action as you push down or up on his or her hands ______________

c. Touching the child's elbow with a vibrating tuning fork ______________________________

2. Identify the seizure described below as psychomotor, absence, tonic-clonic, or simple partial.

a. Generalized seizures with a prodromal, aural, tonic, and clonic stage ______________________

b. Involves only one area of the brain; no altered level of consciousness ______________________

c. May begin with a sudden change in posture, circumoral pallor, a 5-minute loss of consciousness without a postictal stage ______________________

d. "Petit mal," generalized seizures involving a staring spell lasting for a few seconds

____

Multiple-Answer Multiple Choice

Circle the letter(s) corresponding to the appropriate answer(s). Select all that apply.

1. Which of the following would the nurse expect to assess in a child with migraine headaches?
   A. Bilateral pain under both eyes
   B. Pain aggravated by routine activity
   C. Family history of migraine headaches
   D. Report of blurred vision prior to headache
   E. Relief commonly obtained with acetaminophen

CHAPTER 50

Nursing Care of the Child With a Disorder of the Eyes or Ears

CHAPTER OVERVIEW

Chapter 50 discusses the eyes and ears as essential sensory organs. Disorders involving these organs in childhood may retard normal growth and development and, if untreated, may lead to long-term illness. This chapter addresses the structure of the eyes and ears, the physiology of vision and hearing, and common vision and hearing disorders, as well as the nurse's role in health promotion and management of vision and hearing disorders.

LEARNING OBJECTIVES

After mastering the content in this chapter, you should be able to do the following:

1. Describe the structure and function of the eyes and ears and disorders of these organs that affect children.
2. Assess the child who has a disorder of vision or hearing.
3. Formulate nursing diagnoses related to the child with a disorder of vision or hearing.
4. Establish appropriate outcomes for the child with a disorder of vision or hearing.
5. Plan nursing interventions for the child with a disorder of vision or hearing.
6. Implement nursing care to meet the specific needs of the child who has a disorder of the eyes or ears.
7. Evaluate outcomes for achievement and effectiveness of care.
8. Identify National Health Goals related to vision and hearing disorders of children that nurses could be instrumental in helping the nation achieve.
9. Identify areas related to care of children with vision or hearing disorders that could benefit from additional nursing research or application of evidence-based practice.
10. Use critical thinking to analyze ways that nursing care of children with a dysfunction of vision or hearing could be more family-centered.
11. Integrate knowledge of childhood disorders of the eyes or ears with the nursing process to achieve quality maternal and child health nursing care.

KEY TERMS

accommodation
amblyopia
astigmatism
diplopia
enucleation
fovea centralis
goniotomy
hyperopia
light refraction
myopia
myringotomy
nystagmus
orthoptics
ptosis
stereopsis
strabismus
tympanocentesis

■ Mastering the Information

MATCHING

Match the terms in Column I with a definition, example, or related statement from Column II. Place the letter corresponding to the answer in the space provided.

COLUMN I

1. ____Accommodation
2. ____Chalazion
3. ____Dacryostenosis
4. ____Cerumen
5. ____Ptosis
6. ____Blepharitis marginalia
7. ____Amblyopia
8. ____Nystagmus

9. ____Convergence
10. ____Dacryocystitis

COLUMN II

a. Turning of both eyes medially
b. Infection of the eyelid margin
c. Inflammation of the nasolacrimal duct
d. Rapid, irregular eye movements
e. The inability to raise the upper eyelid normally
f. Interruption of the tear flow; blockage of the lacrimal drainage system
g. Chief function of cleaning the external ear
h. Constriction of the pupil as it adjusts from focusing on a distant point to a near point
i. Low-grade granulation tissue tumor of the meibomian or tarsal gland on the eyelid
j. Reduction in vision due to disuse of a structurally normal eye; "lazy eye"

SHORT ANSWER

Supply the missing term or the information requested.

1. ______________ is the ability to locate an object in space relative to other objects.
2. Eye exercises are referred to as ______________.

Applying Your Knowledge

CASE STUDY

Ms. Jones's foster daughter Sally, age 6, was admitted to the hospital for surgery on the left eye. The presurgical diagnosis was a cataract of the left eye. The history and physical examination revealed that Sally's mother is a teenager and Sally has been in foster care since age 2. There was no medical history, and the laboratory and examination report stated that the lens of the left eye was opaque at the edges.

1. What would the nurse suspect as the etiology of the cataract?
2. In this condition would the retina appear red, black, or white?
3. Postoperatively, Sally complains of thirst; the postoperative orders read, "may have fluids when fully awake." When would the nurse allow Sally to have fluids, and why?
4. When teaching Ms. Jones postoperative care, what preventive measures would you want to address?

CRITICAL INQUIRY EXERCISE

1. Prepare an interactive program for a school-age child who is hospitalized for a scheduled eye surgery. Focus on anticipatory guidance, before and after surgery. Incorporate measures to reduce anxiety and promote independence, and use parental participation.
2. Prepare a list of key points for parents to remember when interacting with their school-age child in the hospital environment.

CRITICAL EXPLORATION

1. Make an appointment to visit the local support chapter for citizens who are deaf. Identify the support groups organized in cooperation with this agency. Note the teaching materials and classes made available to support the parents of the child with a hearing disability.
2. Visit a health clinic and participate in the hearing and vision screening for children entering school. Observe the steps taken when a child is found to have a vision or hearing problem.

Practicing for NCLEX

MULTIPLE-CHOICE QUESTIONS

Circle the letter that corresponds to the best answer for each question.

1. The nurse should expect which of the following findings when assessing a child with acute otitis media?
   A. Excessive cerumen in the outer ear
   B. Recent respiratory tract infection
   C. Increased mobility on the pneumatic examination
   D. Copious amount of tenacious fluid

2. The primary cause of visual impairment in children is:
   A. Ocular trauma
   B. Exposure to elevated oxygen levels during infancy
   C. Congenital malformations
   D. Eye infection

3. To visualize the inner surface of a child's lower eyelid and most of the bottom globe, the nurse would:
   A. Pull the top eyelid outward and up
   B. Invert the top eyelid with a special apparatus
   C. Press on the lower lid with a fingertip
   D. Use a cotton-tipped applicator to flip the lower lid

4. If the ciliary body of the eye is involved with a penetration injury, sympathetic iritis may occur. This is described as:
   A. A hemorrhagic paralysis
   B. Inflammation of the opposite eye
   C. A global contusion
   D. An infectious process of the globe

5. The nurse would suspect which of the following in a child is scheduled for tonometry?
   A. Cataracts
   B. Diplopia
   C. Retinal detachment
   D. Glaucoma

6. A child is to undergo a goniotomy procedure to provide an opening to the canal of Schlemm. Preoperatively, which of these drugs would the nurse expect to administer to this child?
   A. Ampicillin (Amoxil)
   B. Cefazolin (Ancef)
   C. Acetazolamide (Diamox)
   D. Atropine

7. Which of the following conditions is likely to occur as a sequela to untreated cataracts in infants?
   A. Amblyopia
   B. Dacryostenosis
   C. Astigmatism
   D. Keratitis

8. Which of the following would be important for the nurse to include in the plan of care for a child who is being prepared to undergo eye surgery?
   A. Showing the child a doll with patches over both eyes
   B. Restraining the child at the wrist bilaterally for 24 hours
   C. Avoiding discussion of the impending surgery
   D. Introducing the child to other children on the unit

ALTERNATE FORMAT QUESTIONS

Fill in the Blank

Supply the missing term or the information requested.

1. ——— is a refractive error (farsightedness) in which vision is blurry at close range.

2. ——— is a congenital incomplete closure of the facial cleft.

Multiple-Answer Multiple Choice

Circle the letter(s) corresponding to the appropriate answer(s). Select all that apply.

1. Which of the following statements about ear disorders is accurate?
   A. In swimmer's ear, Pseudomonas and Candida are often found to be agents involved in the infection.
   B. An internal ear canal altered by a fungal disease may appear brown or black.
   C. There is a higher incidence of otitis media in infants who are breast-fed than in those who are formula-fed.
   D. A myringotomy is a surgical procedure used to drain purulent fluids from an infected middle ear.
   E. The inner ear canal should be cleaned regularly with a cotton-tipped swab to prevent the accumulation of drainage and cerumen.

CHAPTER 51

Nursing Care of the Child With a Musculoskeletal Disorder

CHAPTER OVERVIEW

Chapter 51 discusses the common musculoskeletal disorders experienced in childhood and the potential effects of these disorders on the child's growth and development. The use of the nursing process to plan and provide age-appropriate nursing care addressing the physiologic and psychological needs of the child with musculoskeletal disorders and of family members is explored.

LEARNING OBJECTIVES

After mastering the content in this chapter, you should be able to do the following:

1. Describe common musculoskeletal disorders in children.
2. Assess the child with a musculoskeletal disorder.
3. Use the nursing process to identify and address nursing diagnoses related to the child with a musculoskeletal disorder.
4. Identify National Health Goals related to musculoskeletal disorders and children that nurses can be instrumental in helping the nation achieve.
5. Identify areas related to care of the child with a musculoskeletal disorder that could benefit from additional nursing research.
6. Use critical thinking to analyze ways that care of the child immobilized by a cast or traction can be more family-centered.
7. Synthesize knowledge of musculoskeletal disorders with the nursing process to achieve quality child health nursing care.

KEY TERMS

apposition
arthroscopy
cartilage
diaphysis
distraction
epiphyseal plate
epiphysis
fracture
long bones
malleoli
metaphysis
myopathy
periosteum
petaling
remodeling
reabsorption
sequestrum
smooth muscle
striated muscle
traction

■ Mastering the Information

MATCHING

Match the terms in Column I with a definition, example, or related statement from Column II. Place the letter corresponding to the answer in the space provided.

COLUMN I

1. ____Apposition
2. ____Diaphysis
3. ____Epiphyseal plate
4. ____Genu varum
5. ____Metaphysis
6. ____Metatarsus adductus
7. ____Myopathy
8. ____Osteogenesis imperfecta
9. ____Skeletal traction
10. ____Striated muscle
11. ____Smooth muscle

COLUMN II

a. Acquired or inherited disease of the muscular system
b. The type of muscle responsible for gastrointestinal peristalsis
c. The predominant type of muscle in the body
d. The cartilage segment at which increase in long bone length occurs
e. The thin area between the long bone shaft and the rounded end of the bone
f. The long central shaft of the long bone
g. Evident when there is over an inch between the medial surfaces of the knees when standing with the malleoli of the ankles touching
h. The passing of a pin or wire through the skin into the end of the long bone to immobilize a fracture
i. Application for an infant to allow urine and feces to drain away from a cast
j. The amount of end-to-end contact of the bone fragments
k. Connective tissue disorder characterized by the formation of brittle bones
l. Turning in of the forefoot; can be corrected with stretching exercises

SHORT ANSWER

Supply the missing term or the information requested.

1. A bone injury occurring at the ______ ______ of the long bone may result in irregular or abnormal bone length, and injury to the ______ of the bone may result in irregular bone width.
2. Proper fitting of crutches requires a space of ______ to ______ inches between the axilla crutch pad and the child's axilla and elbow flexion of about ______ degrees.
3. Osgood-Schlatter disease is a ______ and ______ of the tibial tuberosity occurring in children who are athletic and at the ______ or ______ stage of development.
4. Apophysitis occurs most commonly in ______ who are growing rapidly. Pain produced by this condition can be treated by adding a ______ to the shoe heel to reduce tension on the heel cord.
5. To be classified as juvenile rheumatoid arthritis (JRA), symptoms must begin before ______ years of age and last longer than ______ months. The peak incidence occurs at two periods: between ______ and ______ years of age and ______ and ______ years of age.
6. Discuss why a child with a condition requiring a leg brace might have a nursing diagnosis of "Self-esteem disturbance."
7. What nursing measures could be taken to help a school-age child on complete bed rest with traction meet his developmental tasks?
8. Discuss two measures for managing itching underneath a cast and two measures that should not be used.
9. Discuss three exercises used to strengthen the foot arches of a child with flat feet.
10. Compare and contrast the causes of and the treatment for structural and functional scoliosis.
11. Describe the following types of braces and traction and the appropriate use of each: Milwaukee brace, halo traction, Bryant's traction, Buck's traction, skeletal traction.

■ Applying Your Knowledge

CASE STUDY

Evelyn Demark, 10 years old, has osteogenesis imperfecta and is admitted to your unit with a fracture of the right forearm due to an injury in gymnastics class.

1. What would you need to discuss during your teaching session with Evelyn and her parents related to activity choices?
2. How would Evelyn's plan of care differ if she did not have osteogenesis imperfecta?

CRITICAL INQUIRY EXERCISE

1. Write a care plan for a school-age child hospitalized with bilateral leg traction after an accident. Include age-appropriate activities.
2. What safety and development issues would you include in a teaching plan for a 7-month-old with a broken femur due to a fall down the stairs at home?

CRITICAL EXPLORATION

Walk through your home and the home of a friend. Note any circumstances that could represent a danger to a child.

■ Practicing for NCLEX

MULTIPLE-CHOICE QUESTIONS

Circle the letter that corresponds to the best answer for each question.

1. Benji, age 11, has been diagnosed with osteomyelitis after a right leg injury 2 months ago. He and his parents were told he must be admitted to the hospital for treatment. The nurse should explain which of the following to Benji and his parents?
   A. Benji will need to ambulate immediately after surgery, although it may be uncomfortable.
   B. Blood will be drawn for culture to determine the specific medication for treatment of the infection.
   C. Infection control measures are necessary to prevent the spread of this condition to the entire family.
   D. The antibiotic therapy Benji will need must be administered IV and will be complete before discharge.

2. Amy, 3 years old, has been diagnosed with osteogenesis imperfecta. When planning her care, the nurse should consider which of the following?
   A. Active range-of-motion and weight-lifting exercises will be necessary to strengthen weak long bone shafts.
   B. Amy's parents should be encouraged to facilitate her development by not restricting her activities.
   C. Genetic counseling will be appropriate if Amy's condition is congenital or late-occurring.
   D. The treatment for this condition requires lifelong oral intake of calcium supplements.

3. When teaching Sheila, 13 years old, to walk with crutches, the nurse should instruct her to:
   A. Move one crutch forward at a time when using a three-point swing-through gait
   B. Rest the crutch pad on the upper arm to bear her weight on the axilla crutch pad
   C. Carry books and other items in a backpack to keep her hands free
   D. Use a two-point gait when no weight bearing is allowed

4. Marla, age 12, has a cast on her left leg. During a follow-up phone call, Marla states she is experiencing occasional numbness in her left foot and the foot feels cool. The nurse should respond in which of the following ways?
   A. Explain to Marla that she needs to wiggle her toes frequently to prevent the return of the numbness and coolness.
   B. Inform Marla and her mother of the need to elevate the extremity to promote good circulation.
   C. Instruct Marla and her mother to return to the doctor for possible removal of the cast.
   D. Teach Marla isometric exercises to use when numbness and coolness occur.

5. The nurse would determine that the plan of care for a child with juvenile rheumatoid arthritis (JRA) had been effective if which of the following findings was noted?
   A. The parents state the need to avoid aspirin administration to prevent Reye's syndrome.
   B. Meals are offered after periods of rest and administration of pain medication and are 80% eaten.
   C. Splints are applied during the day and removed at night by parents to promote sleep.
   D. Ice baths are applied to the affected joints by parents twice daily.

6. A care plan for a girl suspected of having myasthenia gravis may include which of the following?
   A. Administering cholinergic drugs to suppress the hyperactivity actions of acetylcholine
   B. Inquiring if the child has had trouble in school recently due to difficulty reading or seeing the board
   C. Reassuring the adolescent female that myasthenia gravis will not affect her childbearing potential
   D. Scheduling medications after mealtime to decrease gastrointestinal symptoms, choking, and possible aspiration

7. Congenital muscular dystrophy differs from Duchenne's disease and facioscapulohumeral muscular dystrophy in which of the following ways?
   A. Congenital muscular dystrophy results in degeneration of muscle fibers.
   B. Congenital muscular dystrophy can result in problems with parental bonding.
   C. In facioscapulohumeral muscular dystrophy, the predominant symptom is facial weakness.
   D. Victims of Duchenne's disease and their families should have genetic counseling.

ALTERNATE FORMAT QUESTIONS

Fill in the Blank

Supply the missing term or the information requested.

1. During the periods of acute inflammation in JRA, joints should be _______, but children may do ______________________________ exercise.
2. A ________ is a muscle-tendon injury; a _____ is a ligament injury.

Multiple-Answer Multiple Choice

Circle the letter(s) corresponding to the appropriate answer(s). Select all that apply.

1. Which are appropriate nursing interventions for the child undergoing spinal instrumentation for treatment of scoliosis?
   A. Maintain the head of the bed at a 45-degree elevation.
   B. Logroll the child to a side-lying position every 2 hours unless Luque/segmented rods are used.
   C. Monitor the neurologic and vascular function of the extremities every hour for the first 24 hours.
   D. Explain the need to keep the child NPO until bowel sounds are audible.
   E. Instruct the parents not to touch the child during the early postoperative period.
   F. Reassure the child that although the rods usually remain in place permanently, they are not obvious to others.
   G. Instruct the child that good posture is mandatory and to bend at the knees to remove objects from the floor.
   H. Reassure the child that moderate movement is safe after final cast removal following rod insertion.
   I. Explain to parents that even severe scoliosis can be completely corrected with surgery.
   J. Inform female clients with scoliosis that childbearing is contraindicated.

CHAPTER 52

Nursing Care of the Child With a Traumatic Injury

CHAPTER OVERVIEW

Accidents are a major cause of childhood morbidity and mortality, and prevention is a goal that nurses and other health care providers always strive for. However, not all accidents can be prevented. Chapter 52 describes the principles of nursing care for the child with a traumatic injury. The uses of the nursing process to assess, plan, and provide appropriate nursing care and to address the physiologic and psychological needs of the child and family involved with traumatic injury are discussed.

LEARNING OBJECTIVES

After mastering the content in this chapter, you should be able to do the following:

1. Describe the causes and consequences of common accidents and injuries in childhood, as well as measures to prevent them.
2. Assess a child injured from an accident such as poisoning or burning.
3. Use the nursing process to identify and address nursing diagnoses related to the injured child.
4. Identify National Health Goals related to children and trauma that nurses can be instrumental in helping the nation achieve.
5. Use critical thinking to analyze ways that accidents and injuries can be prevented in childhood.
6. Synthesize knowledge of injuries in childhood with the nursing process to achieve quality child health nursing care.

KEY TERMS

allografting
autografting
contrecoup injury
debridement
drowning
escharotomy
heterografts
homografting
near-drowning
otorrhea
plumbism
rhinorrhea
stupor

■ Mastering the Information

MATCHING

Match the terms in Column I with a definition, example, or related statement from Column II. Place the letter corresponding to the answer in the space provided.

COLUMN I

1. ____Allografting
2. ____Chelating agents
3. ____Contrecoup injury
4. ____Contusion
5. ____Escharotomy
6. ____Heterografting
7. ____Leptomeningeal cyst
8. ____Plumbism
9. ____Rhinorrhea
10. ____Stupor
11. ____Autografting

COLUMN II

a. Cutting into the tough leathery scab over a burned area to release a tight band around an extremity

b. Placing of skin from cadavers or a donor on a cleaned burn site

c. A tearing or laceration of brain tissue, with symptoms specific to the brain area affected

d. Grogginess from which an individual can be roused

e. Lead poisoning; usually occurs in toddlers and preschool children

f. Clear fluid draining from the nose; if it is cerebrospinal fluid it will be positive for glucose

g. A concussion on the side of the brain opposite that which was struck; occurs as the brain recoils from the force of the blow

h. Skin from a nonhuman source, such as porcine (pig), used to promote skin growth after a burn

i. Skin taken from an unburned area of a burn victim's body and placed on a prepared burned area to facilitate healing

j. Substances that act to remove lead from soft tissue and bone and eliminate it in the urine

k. Results from projection of the arachnoid membrane into the fracture site; may cause symptoms of increased intracranial pressure

SHORT ANSWER

Supply the missing term or the information requested.

1. The extent of a child's injury depends on ______, ______, and ______.
2. The Glasgow Coma Scale includes assessment of ______ ______, responses to speech and pain, and ______ and ______ responses.
3. Nurses can help the nation meet health goals concerned with trauma by being ______ care providers who provide counseling on ______ ______ to parents and ______.
4. Discuss the appropriate method for discharge teaching of parents of injured children discharged from the emergency room.
5. Explain why the "rule of nines" cannot be used to determine the extent of burns on infants and children.
6. Discuss the reason burn injuries to the face and throat can be more hazardous than other burn injuries.
7. Describe the infection control measures used for burn victims.
8. Describe the appropriate emergency treatment for the indicated burn injuries: first-degree; second- and third-degree; electrical burn; facial or neck burns.

▪ Applying Your Knowledge

CASE STUDY

Mr. and Mrs. Chin come to your emergency room with their 3-year-old son, Jay. Jay is an active child who has broken his arm and sprained a wrist climbing on furniture. Jay likes to ride his tricycle around the house and yard and once nearly drank a liquid cleaner that was not placed out of reach in the kitchen. Jay's arm is placed in a cast.

1. What psychological supports would you need to provide for Jay and his parents to help them cope with the current injury and plan for Jay's continued development?
2. What safety issues would you need to address with the Chin family, and what further assessments would you make?
3. What age-appropriate activities would you suggest to the Chin family to facilitate Jay's development?

CRITICAL INQUIRY EXERCISE

1. What safety suggestions could you give to a couple who have open fireplaces and space heaters in their home and three active children ages 18 months, 3 years, and 5 years?
2. Prepare a plan of care addressing outdoor summer activities and dress for parents of a child who lives on a ranch in the Southwest.

CRITICAL EXPLORATION

1. Visit a burn center and observe the care measures taken for clients at various ages and with various types and degrees of burns.

2. Locate the names and phone numbers of the emergency medical system and the poison control center in your neighborhood.

■ Practicing for NCLEX

MULTIPLE-CHOICE QUESTIONS

Circle the letter that corresponds to the best answer for each question.

1. Which of the following would be a serious danger sign if noted in a child after head trauma?
   A. Complaint of headache along the area of trauma
   B. Blood pressure moving from 120/80 to 130/50
   C. Memory deficit with inability to recall time or date
   D. Pupils equal and briskly reactive to light

2. Care of the child in a coma would include:
   A. Encouraging parents to be positive, since coma is often short term in children
   B. Performing passive range-of-motion exercises to maintain muscle tone
   C. Feeding the child with a spoon and fork to stimulate memories of normal activity
   D. Maintaining the child in a flat, supine position to simulate normal sleeping position

3. Jan, age 13, is admitted with third-degree burns over 25% of her body. Which of the following is an immediate concern in Jan's plan of care?
   A. Liberal medication to control Jan's severe pain
   B. Arranging age-appropriate diversional activities
   C. Preventing hypovolemia and circulatory collapse
   D. Increasing oral intake of proteins to build tissue

4. A realistic outcome criterion for the parents of a child who is the victim of traumatic injury would be for the parents to:
   A. Admit responsibility for the child's trauma
   B. Allow the child to perform household chores without supervision to strengthen self-esteem
   C. Prevent all future accidental childhood injury
   D. State measures they can take to prevent common accidents from occurring

ALTERNATE FORMAT QUESTIONS

Fill in the Blank

Supply the missing term or the information requested.

1. Full-thickness or ______ degree burns are not extremely painful.

2. Equipment used to care for a severely burned child must be ____________ to prevent wound infection.

3. Second- or third-degree burns may receive ____________ treatment, which involves leaving the burned area exposed to air.

Multiple-Answer Multiple Choice

Circle the letter(s) corresponding to the appropriate answer(s). Select all that apply.

1. Select the appropriate intervention(s) for the conditions listed.
   A. Subdural hematoma: Monitor for seizures, vomiting, or hyperirritability for up to 20 days after the trauma.
   B. Acetaminophen poisoning: Administer syrup of ipecac followed by acetylcysteine/Mucomyst in a carbonated drink.
   C. Caustic poisoning: Administer syrup of ipecac followed by cold water or milk.
   D. Hydrocarbon ingestion: Monitor the child for respiratory irritation.
   E. Iron poisoning: Monitor for initial nausea, diarrhea, and abdominal pain followed by melena and hematemesis and shock 12 hours later.
   F. Lead poisoning: Instruct parents to repaint the home before the child is discharged.
   G. Plant poisoning: Reassure parents that this is not serious and requires no treatment.
   H. Recreational drug poisoning: Attempt to determine if the ingestion was a suicide attempt if the child is over 7 years of age.

2. Select the appropriate intervention(s) for the conditions listed.
   A. Concussion: Instruct parents not to allow the child to sleep for 24 hours after the trauma.
   B. Foreign body obstruction: Irrigate the child's ear canal with saline to remove a peanut.
   C. Frostbite: Place the affected body part in hot water to restore circulation immediately.
   D. Snake bite: Apply a cold compress to the site immediately and keep the site in a dependent position to slow venom spread; monitor for bruising and bleeding.
   E. Facial burn: Monitor for stridor or other signs of respiratory tract obstruction.
   F. Third-degree burn over 10% of the body: Decrease fluid intake to aid kidneys in filtration of waste and concentration of urine.
   G. Any traumatic injury: Restrict parental involvement in care of the child to decrease demands on parents.

CHAPTER 53

Nursing Care of the Child with Cancer

CHAPTER OVERVIEW

The diagnosis of cancer in a child can be devastating to a family. However, the prognosis for children with cancer is continually improving. Chapter 53 provides an overview of the special care needs of the child with cancer. The physical and psychological effects of various types of childhood cancers are discussed. The use of the nursing process to plan and provide care for the child and the family coping with cancer is explored.

LEARNING OBJECTIVES

After mastering the content in this chapter, you should be able to do the following:

1. Define terms related to tumor growth such as neoplasm, benign, malignant, sarcoma, and carcinoma, and describe normal cell growth and theories that explain how cells are altered to become neoplastic in children.
2. Assess the child with a neoplastic process such as a rhabdomyosarcoma, neuroblastoma, Wilms' tumor, or leukemia.
3. Use the nursing process to identify and address nursing diagnoses related to the child with a malignancy.
4. Identify National Health Goals related to children and cancer that nurses can be instrumental in helping the nation achieve.
5. Use critical thinking to analyze ways that nursing care for the child with a neoplasm can be more family-centered.
6. Synthesize knowledge of abnormal cell growth in children with the nursing process to achieve quality child health nursing care.

KEY TERMS

biopsy
chemotherapeutic agent
Ewing's sarcoma
leukemia
lymphoma
metastasis
neoplasm
neuroblastoma
oncogenic virus
oncogenic virus
osteogenic sarcoma
rhabdomyosarcoma
sarcoma
tumor staging

■ Mastering the Information

MATCHING

Match the terms in Column I with a definition, example, or related statement from Column II. Place the letter corresponding to the answer in the space provided.

COLUMN I

1. ____Alopecia
2. ____Allogeneic
3. ____Astrocytoma
4. ____Medulloblastoma
5. ____Neoplasm
6. ____Neuroblastoma
7. ____Oncogenic
8. ____Osteogenic sarcoma
9. ____Rhabdomyosarcoma
10. ____Staging

COLUMN II

a. A term commonly used for a new abnormal growth that does not respond to growth control mechanisms
b. Cancer-causing agent
c. Hair loss; occurs secondary to almost all chemotherapeutic cancer drugs
d. A transplant between a histocompatible person and a child with cancer
e. Designating the extent of a malignant process
f. Slow-growing cystic tumor arising from the glial tissue of the neural cells
g. Fast-growing tumor found most commonly in the cerebellum
h. A tumor of striated muscle
i. A tumor arising from the cells of the sympathetic nervous system
j. A malignant tumor of long bone involving rapidly growing bone tissue

SHORT ANSWER

Supply the missing term or the information requested.

1. Because cells lining the stomach are fast-growing, ——— and ——— are common side effects of chemotherapy.
2. Chemotherapy for acute lymphatic leukemia is given first in a ——— phase, next in a ——— phase, and finally in a ——————— phase.
3. Early symptoms in children with leukemia are —————, —————, and —————.
4. Hodgkin's disease is confirmed by biopsies of the ————— ————— and ————— .
5. An adolescent with osteosarcoma who must undergo leg amputation might achieve the goal of realizing the amputation is ——— to save ——— —————————————————.
6. Neuroblastomas may cause loss of motor function due to ——— on the spinal nerves or ——— into the intervertebral foramina.
7. Describe five of the common categories of chemotherapeutic cancer agents.
8. Discuss factors that may contribute to decreased nutritional status in a child with cancer.

Applying Your Knowledge

CASE STUDY

Mr. and Mrs. Morrell have been advised that Joseph has a brain tumor. He was admitted 2 days ago for preoperative lab work. Today is the day of the surgery, and you are assigned as Joseph's operating room nurse. When reading the surgical checklist, you found that Joseph had not received an enema or any methods to evacuate the bowel.

1. What would be your response after learning of this situation?
2. Provide a rationale for each of these postoperative orders for Joseph: NPO, keep HOB elevated 45 degrees, position on side, administer eye drops q4h, neuro checks q2h, change dressing when wet, monitor vital signs, D5 1/4 NS to KVO.

CRITICAL INQUIRY EXERCISE

1. Prepare a teaching plan for a child with a diagnosis of leukemia or her parents.
2. Develop a tool to contrast the presenting symptoms that may be seen on an assessment for a child presenting with leukemia. The tool should help you determine the type of malignancy based on the clinical picture.

CRITICAL EXPLORATION

Visit a pediatric cancer ward. Note the varied types of childhood cancer and the types of medical and nursing treatments being provided.

Practicing for NCLEX

MULTIPLE-CHOICE QUESTIONS

Circle the letter that corresponds to the best answer for each question.

1. Mrs. Peters states she's glad her son Tim's cancer was caught early and now he is safe from cancer in later life. The nurse should respond with which of the following principles in mind?
   A. Cancer is less likely to strike Tim again.
   B. Childhood cancer usually instills an immunity to cancer.
   C. Children surviving one cancer have a greater risk for a second cancer.
   D. Cancer onset is unpredictable and carries no pattern of recurrence.

2. Children with cancer would be most vulnerable for skeletal side effects from radiation therapy at which of the following ages?
   A. 2 years
   B. 4 years
   C. 6 years
   D. 12 years

3. Which of the following is true about radiation therapy?
   A. The skin areas at which the radiotherapy is directed should be washed daily with soap and water.
   B. Creams and lotions should not be applied to the radiation site until a radiation series is complete.
   C. Sedatives and analgesics should be withheld during radiotherapy.
   D. Radiation may result in excessive salivary gland function.

4. Which of the following nursing interventions is most important when caring for a child receiving vincristine?
   A. Administering salicylates to relieve nerve pain
   B. Encouraging intake of high-fiber foods
   C. Monitoring for frequent diarrheal stools
   D. Planning age-appropriate coloring or drawing activities

5. The decreased platelet production from leukemia's effect on a child's bone marrow would result in which of the following symptoms?
   A. Flushed skin
   B. Epistaxis
   C. Hyperthermia
   D. Tachycardia

6. Children who have a brain tumor will have which of the following symptoms?
   A. Abdominal pain
   B. Diarrhea
   C. Hypotension
   D. Vomiting

7. Which of the following interventions may be needed for the parents of a child diagnosed with a brain tumor?
   A. Allowing the parents to delay treatment for weeks if needed until the denial stage resolves
   B. Explaining that removal of a small peripheral tumor is a minor surgical procedure
   C. Reinforcing preoperative explanations about the nature of the child's diagnosis after surgery is over
   D. Reassuring parents that radiation and chemotherapy can cure brain tumors and prevent metastasis

ALTERNATE FORMAT QUESTIONS

Fill in the Blank

Supply the missing term or the information requested.

1. ________ ________ is a malignant tumor occurring most often in the bone marrow of the midshaft of long bones.
2. ________ is a rare malignant tumor of the eye.
3. ________ may be required for a large malignant tumor of the eye.

Multiple-Answer Multiple Choice

Circle the letter(s) corresponding to the appropriate answer(s). Select all that apply.

1. Select the appropriate interventions for nursing care for a child with cancer.
   A. Encouraging children receiving chemotherapy to take clear fluids, even if they are nauseated, to prevent uric acid buildup in the kidney
   B. Using ice packs to the scalp of children with leukemia to decrease alopecia
   C. Placing a child receiving immunosuppressive drugs on wound and skin isolation to minimize spread of infection
   D. Placing a warm compress on a site of infiltration of a chemotherapeutic agent
   E. Administering live virus vaccines to immunosuppressed children to achieve maximum protection against infection
   F. Pushing fluids with children receiving chemotherapy to reduce loss of kidney function
   G. Monitoring a child receiving chemotherapy for leukemia for nuchal rigidity, headache, irritability, and vomiting
   H. Encouraging normal activity and regular school for children in the maintenance phase of leukemia therapy
   I. Reassuring the parents of a child having surgery for removal of a brain tumor that the child will be awake and oriented after surgery

UNIT IX

The Nursing Role in Restoring and Maintaining the Health of Children and Families With Mental Health Disorders

CHAPTER 54

Nursing Care of the Child with a Cognitive or Mental Health Disorder

CHAPTER OVERVIEW

Children who are cognitively impaired have the same fundamental needs as other children. The nurse has a responsibility to provide the families of these children with skills to observe, solve problems, make decisions, and prevent illness. This chapter presents common illnesses, identifies behaviors, and explores methods of helping the family manage.

LEARNING OBJECTIVES

After mastering the content in this chapter, you should be able to do the following:

1. Describe common cognitive and mental health disorders in children.
2. Assess a child for a cognitive or mental health disorder.
3. Formulate nursing diagnoses related to the cognitive or mental health disorders of childhood.
4. Establish appropriate outcomes for the child with a cognitive or mental health disorder.
5. Plan nursing care for the child with a cognitive or mental health disorder.
6. Implement nursing care for the child with a cognitive or mental health disorder.
7. Evaluate outcomes for achievement and effectiveness of care.
8. Identify National Health Goals related to cognitive or mental health disorders that nurses can be instrumental in helping the nation achieve.
9. Identify areas related to cognitive or mental health that could benefit from additional nursing research or application of evidence-based practice.
10. Analyze ways that care of the child with a cognitive or mental health disorder can be more family-centered.
11. Integrate knowledge of childhood cognitive and mental health disorders and the nursing process to achieve quality maternal and child health nursing care.

KEY TERMS

anhedonia
binge eating
catatonia
choreiform movements
complex vocal tics
coprolalia
dyslexia
echolalia
expressed emotion
flat affect
graphesthesia
hyperactivity
labile mood
motor tics
palilalia
purging
school phobia
stereognosis
vocal tics

▪ Mastering the Information

MATCHING

Match the terms in Column I with a definition, example, or related statement from Column II. Place the letter corresponding to the answer in the space provided.

COLUMN I

1. _____Encopresis
2. _____Motor tics
3. _____Catatonia
4. _____Dyslexia
5. _____Tourette's disease

COLUMN II

a. Muscle movements such as rapid repetitive eye blinking or facial twitching
b. Inherited syndrome of facial and complex vocal tics
c. Passing feces in culturally unacceptable places
d. A learning disorder involving a reading disability
e. Behaviors seen in children with schizophrenia, characterized by withdrawal and stuporous depression

SHORT ANSWER

Supply the missing term or the information requested.

1. List the criteria for mental retardation as described by DSM-IV-TR.
2. Define labile mood.
3. Describe graphesthesia, stereognosis, and choreiform movements.
4. Children with schizophrenia may reveal what type of affect?

■ Applying Your Knowledge

CASE STUDY

Stephen is 2.5 years old; his mother brings him to the health clinic with an ear infection. The history and physical exam reveal that Stephen's behavior is quite different from that of the other siblings. The mother reports that he hates to be held, utters sounds only when trying to talk, gets upset easily, and screams constantly. You notice that Stephen has excoriated lesions on his thumbs.

1. Based on the information, what would be a probable diagnosis for Stephen?
2. What type of temperament is usually seen with these children?
3. How can the nurse assist the parents in bonding with Stephen and providing developmental support?

CRITICAL INQUIRY EXERCISE

1. Arrange with your instructor to invite to your classroom the mother of an 8-year-old or older child with a cognitive or mental health disorder. Ask her to explain how she prepares the child for health visits and what she does in the household to protect the child from injury.
2. Develop an assessment tool to be used in a clinical setting to help the health care professional recognize the signs and symptoms of teenage depression.

CRITICAL EXPLORATION

Attend a school that has an academic or vocational curriculum for the retarded student. Research the activities in the curriculum that will help the student become a functional member of his or her community and society.

■ Practicing for NCLEX

MULTIPLE-CHOICE QUESTIONS

Circle the letter that corresponds to the best answer for each question.

1. After teaching the parents of a child diagnosed with ADHD about the disorder, the nurse determines that teaching has been successful if the parents identify which of the following as a characteristic of this disorder?
   A. Hypoactivity
   B. Attentiveness
   C. Impulsiveness
   D. Conscientiousness

2. When providing anticipatory guidance to parents of a hyperactive child, the nurse would encourage them to:
   A. Assign chores appropriate to the child's age
   B. Be flexible and lenient regarding limits
   C. Give instructions to this child in the group setting with the other siblings
   D. Delay punishing the child to allow the child time to think about mistakes

3. Baby girl Franshon, 12 months old, is admitted to the hospital for electrolyte imbalance and to rule intestinal obstruction. After careful assessment it is determined that Baby Franshon is regurgitating her food after ingestion and then reswallowing it. Research postulates that this is a form of self-stimulation by the infant termed:
   A. Encopresis
   B. Rumination
   C. Anhedonia
   D. Bulimia

4. Felicia is 15 years old and is admitted to the hospital with anorexia nervosa. She is a model and often spoken of as an overachiever. As the nurse interviews Felicia and her family, she may discover other findings such as:
   A. Early development of secondary sex characteristics
   B. Permissive parenting
   C. Amenorrhea
   D. Hyperglycemia

5. Which of the following is commonly seen in children with anorexia nervosa?
   A. Morbid obesity
   B. Ingesting copious amounts of water
   C. Body mass index above 85% of expected
   D. Binge eating and purging

6. A child with an IQ of 44 would be categorized as having which type of mental retardation?
   A. Mild
   B. Moderate
   C. Severe
   D. Profound

ALTERNATE FORMAT QUESTIONS

Fill in the Blank

Supply the missing term or the information requested.

1. ——— is the term that describes the eating of nonfood substances such as dirt, clay, and crayons.
2. ——— disorder is a perplexing condition that parents may view as the child rejecting them.

Multiple-Answer Multiple Choice

Circle the letter(s) corresponding to the appropriate answer(s). Select all that apply.

1. Which of the following statement(s) about bulimia nervosa are correct?
   A. Girls with bulimia may be slightly underweight or at normal weight.
   B. Purgatives, laxatives, and diuretics are used to control weight.
   C. Counseling focuses on having the girl relinquish control.
   D. Erosion of tooth enamel from vomiting occurs less frequently.
   E. The individual with bulimia views food as revolting.

CHAPTER 55

Nursing Care of the Family in Crisis: Abuse and Violence in the Family

CHAPTER OVERVIEW

Child and domestic abuse is a national problem with serious consequences for children. Chapter 55 describes the physiologic and psychological effects of child and domestic abuse. The use of the nursing process to identify, plan, and provide appropriate nursing care to help victims and their family members or significant others cope with the trauma of child and domestic abuse is discussed.

LEARNING OBJECTIVES

After mastering the content in this chapter, you should be able to do the following:

1. Discuss the types of abuse seen in families and the theories explaining them.
2. Assess a physically or emotionally abused family.
3. Use the nursing process to identify and address nursing diagnoses related to the abused family.
4. Identify National Health Goals related to child abuse that nurses can be instrumental in helping the nation achieve.
5. Identify areas related to care of the abused child that could benefit from additional nursing research.
6. Use critical thinking to analyze ways that nurses can be instrumental in preventing child abuse.
7. Synthesize knowledge of family abuse with the nursing process to achieve quality child health nursing care.

KEY TERMS

abuse
disorganization phase
failure to thrive
incest
intimate partner abuse
learned helplessness
mandatory reporters
molestation
Munchausen syndrome by proxy
pedophile
permissive reporters
rape trauma syndrome
reorganization syndrome
shaken baby syndrome
silent rape syndrome

■ Mastering the Information

MATCHING

Match the terms in Column I with a definition, example, or related statement from Column II. Place the letter corresponding to the answer in the space provided.

COLUMN I

1. ____Abuse
2. ____Disorganization phase
3. ____Incest
4. ____Mandatory reporters
5. ____Molestation
6. ____Munchausen syndrome by proxy
7. ____Pedophile
8. ____Failure to thrive
9. ____Shaken baby syndrome
10. ____Reorganization phase

COLUMN II

a. Severe activity between family members
b. A form of child neglect occurring due to a disturbance in the parent–child relationship
c. Parents who repeatedly bring a child to a health care facility reporting symptoms of illness when, in fact, the child is well
d. Willful injury of one person by another
e. The first stage of rape trauma syndrome; lasts about 3 days
f. The second stage of rape trauma syndrome; may last months or years
g. People who must notify the authorities of suspected abuse; nurses fall into this category
h. Sexual involvement between an adult and child, such as oral–genital contact or viewing genitals
i. An adult who seeks out children for sexual gratification
j. Whiplash injury to the neck, edema to the brain stem, retinal hemorrhages, and potential respiratory arrest

SHORT ANSWER

Supply the missing term or the information requested.

1. The triad of circumstances that generally combine to result in child abuse are a ________ ________, a child seen as ________ in the parent's eyes, and a ________ ________ or circumstance.
2. Discuss why children in an abusive family situation might have other undiagnosed medical problems.
3. Discuss one major reason why victims of child abuse might grow to be abusers themselves.
4. Why should a nurse examine his or her personal feelings related to the abuser and the victim in a domestic abuse situation?
5. Discuss one method of differentiating between organic and nonorganic failure to thrive.
6. List symptoms of infants demonstrating failure to thrive relative to physical and social development.

■ Applying Your Knowledge

CASE STUDY

Alissa, age 26, appears in your emergency room with her 4-year-old daughter, Daisy. She states, "He's hurting her. See, he's made her bleed." Alissa is pointing at Daisy's underpants, which are soiled with a dark-red stain.

1. What would your initial actions be?
2. How would you proceed in your care planning for Daisy?
3. What issues might you need to address with Alissa if the "he" she referred to was Alissa's husband or live-in boyfriend? If "he" is Alissa's father (Daisy's grandfather)?

CRITICAL INQUIRY EXERCISE

1. Describe your feelings about a report of rape made by a female child 5 years of age who says, "Daddy hurt me."
2. What would your response be to a male adolescent who reports that his coach sexually abused him, or to a wife who says her husband raped her?

CRITICAL EXPLORATION

Visit a rape crisis center in your neighborhood. Note three activities performed by the nurse in that setting.

■ Practicing for NCLEX

MULTIPLE-CHOICE QUESTIONS

Circle the letter that corresponds to the best answer for each question.

1. Because abuse involves and affects all the members of a family, the nurse should have which of the following as part of the care plan goals?
   A. Disrupting the dysfunctional family
   B. Improving overall family functioning
   C. Punishing the abusive family member
   D. Removing the abuse victim from the family

2. When planning a strategy to address child and domestic abuse, the nurse should do which of the following?
   A. Lecture parents suspected of child abuse on the evils of violence.
   B. Report suspected child abuse whenever a child with bruises is admitted.
   C. Stop parental visitation immediately if child abuse is suspected.
   D. Work with pregnant teen groups to teach parenting skills.

3. At his first physical, Bob, 14 years old, stated that the multiple long whip-like scars on his back occurred as a result of falling backward against a rough bedroom floor when he was playing with a friend. The nurse should respond in which of the following ways?
   A. Ask additional questions regarding the cause of the injury and any other injuries noted.
   B. Discuss with Bob the fact that his clumsiness is probably a part of his adolescence and that he will outgrow it.
   C. Instruct Bob in the importance of exercise and good nutrition to avoid easy bruising.
   D. Tell Bob you do not believe him and you want to know if his parents caused his injuries.

4. Sheila, 11 years old, is admitted with vaginal bleeding. The nurse notices that Sheila and her mother are very nervous but state that they are "sure it's just menstrual blood." The nurse should initially do which of the following?
   A. Accept the fact that Sheila is probably beginning menses; don't jump to conclusions.
   B. Explain to Sheila and her mother that menstrual bleeding does not occur at this early age.
   C. Insist that Sheila's mother tell if someone is abusing Sheila.
   D. Gently examine Sheila for torn perineal tissue or lacerations.

5. Which of the following would place a parent at high risk for being a child abuser?
   A. Being poor and a member of a minority group
   B. Choosing to have a baby without being married
   C. Having less than a high school education
   D. Severe disappointment with the sex of a new baby

6. Daryl, age 7, states he can't tell about his father's beating him because the beating will get worse. The nurse should remember which of the following when replying to Daryl?
   A. Daryl might be angry with his parents and making up this story.
   B. Daryl's mother can protect him from the father if necessary.
   C. Most institutions can hold a child for 72 hours for protection.
   D. Seven-year-olds are not reliable witnesses of child abuse.

7. A realistic outcome criterion for a woman admitted with a broken collarbone caused by a husband with a history of violence would be that the woman might do which of the following?
   A. Fight back the next time he hurts her.
   B. Identify what she does that causes her husband to become violent.
   C. Leave the abusive man immediately and never see him again.
   D. State the names of two shelters she can go to when necessary.

8. The nurse caring for an abused child or abused woman should do which of the following?
   A. Allow the family members to remain alone together as much as possible, regardless of the situation, to facilitate family stability.
   B. Assume that the abuse was malicious and isolate the victim from family members.
   C. Refrain from becoming emotionally involved in the situation.
   D. Stay with the child or abused woman throughout the examination process and questioning sessions to offer needed support.

9. Which of the following is true about abuse?
   A. Neglect can be an unintentional form of child abuse.
   B. Psychological abuse is not as damaging as physical abuse.
   C. The goal of nursing care in abuse situations is to keep families together throughout therapy.
   D. Victims of abuse experience guilt only if they caused the abuser to become violent.

ALTERNATE FORMAT QUESTIONS

Fill in the Blank

Supply the missing term or the information requested.

1. ——— is often the first person to identify the symptoms of possible child abuse.
2. Excessive use of ——— by the abusive person is strongly associated with abuse.
3. When questioned about an injury, an abused child will usually ——— the parent's story.

Multiple-Answer Multiple Choice

Circle the letter(s) corresponding to the appropriate answer(s). Select all that apply.

1. Select the appropriate interventions for a patient with abuse or violence in the family.
   A. Inform the parents you suspect child abuse as soon as you note suspicious signs.
   B. Interview the victim in front of the abuser to make the abuser confess to the crime.
   C. Examine the child or suspected victim in a fully undressed state whenever possible.
   D. Protect the child's or victim's modesty as much as possible.
   E. Do not try to nurture the infant with failure to thrive since this will interfere with family–child bonding.
   F. Take photographs of injuries and bruises.
   G. Suspect overprotective partners of rape victims of being potential abusers.
   H. Write the exact words spoken by abuse victims and others describing the situation in the patient care chart.
   I. Encourage victims to talk about the abuse or rape to help them begin to work through it.
   J. Instruct women that the examination after the rape will be the only one she will have to submit to.

CHAPTER 56

Nursing Care of the Family Coping With Long-Term or Terminal Illness

CHAPTER OVERVIEW

Chapter 56 discusses the physiologic and emotional concerns related to caring for a family coping with a long-term or fatal illness. The emotional effects of chronic and terminal illness on the entire family as well as on the nursing care provider are reviewed. The use of the nursing process to plan and provide care for the family involved with long-term or terminal illness is explored.

LEARNING OBJECTIVES

After mastering the content in this chapter, you should be able to do the following:

1. Describe common concerns of parents of children with a long-term or fatal illness.
2. Assess adjustment of the child and family with a long-term or terminal illness.
3. Use the nursing process to identify and address nursing diagnoses for the child with a chronic or fatal illness.
4. Identify National Health Goals related to children with long-term or fatal illnesses that nurses could be instrumental in helping the nation achieve.
5. Use critical thinking to analyze ways that nursing care of chronically ill or dying children can be more family-centered.
6. Synthesize knowledge of long-term and fatal illness in children with the nursing process to achieve quality child health nursing care.

KEY TERMS

anticipatory grief
death
grief process
vulnerable children

■ Mastering the Information

MATCHING

Match the terms in Column I with a definition, example, or related statement from Column II. Place the letter corresponding to the answer in the space provided.

COLUMN I

1. _____Infant
2. _____Toddler
3. _____Preschooler
4. _____School-ager
5. _____Adolescent

COLUMN II

A. View death as temporary early in this stage; later realize death is final; focus on how they will cope without parents
B. See death as sleep and fear separation more than death
C. Have no understanding of their impending death; comfort and security are their main focus
D. Have adult concerns of death but view themselves as basically indestructible; need to remain as active as possible
E. May have viewed the death of a relative but do not understand or relate this to their own death; need to maintain routines

COLUMN I

1. ____Anticipatory grief
2. ____Bargaining stage
3. ____Depression
4. ____Denial stage
5. ____Anger stage
6. ____Hospice
7. ____Death
8. ____Organ donation
9. ____Autopsy
10. ____Grief reaction

COLUMN II

A. Absence of respirations, no heart sounds, absence of body movement or reflexes, and dilated fixed pupils

B. The experience that occurs when news of chronic illness or impending death is received

C. Action that may provide a comfort for parents to know a part of their child has helped another child to live

D. Parents may promise to do good deeds so the terminally ill child will get well

E. Parental problem-solving skills are impaired, possibly leading nurse to be ineffective

F. Mandatory if homicide, suicide, or harmful death is suspected

G. A third opinion regarding the disease or prognosis may be requested

H. Option for children allowing them to die in a homelike setting

I. Parents beginning to really think about the child's impending death

J. Parents possibly criticizing the nurse or scolding the child frequently

SHORT ANSWER

Supply the missing term or the information requested.

1. People cope with situations depending on ———, ——————————, and ——————————.
2. A client or family's ability to use health care resources depends on ————— —————, —————, —————, —————, and —————.
3. Two of the reactions a nurse may have to the terminal illness of a child are ——— and ———.
4. Nurses can help the nation meet National Health Goals related to chronic illness in children by educating women to seek care for themselves during pregnancy so ——— ——— are reduced, and seek ——— for their children so diseases that can lead to long-term disability can be prevented.
5. Briefly compare the effects a chronic illness such as diabetes might have on a family with the effects of a chronic illness such as muscular dystrophy.
6. Discuss how the age of the parents might affect their ability to care for a disabled child.
7. Why would healthy parents of a chronically ill or disabled child need to have a will prepared?
8. How might evaluating the plan of care for a family with a terminal child after the child's death be beneficial for a nurse?
9. List three of the seven approaches to communicating with dying children.

■ Applying Your Knowledge

CASE STUDY

Patricia, age 10, is involved in an automobile accident that results in facial scarring. Her parents arrived an hour ago and have been told that plastic surgery will help but cannot fully repair the damage to Patricia's face.

1. What reactions might you expect from Patricia when she discovers the condition of her face? What factors might affect the extent and demonstration of her grief?
2. How might Patricia's reaction differ from that of a 14- or 15-year-old girl?

CRITICAL INQUIRY EXERCISE

1. How might you feel if a patient you cared for over several weeks died on your day off? How would those feelings differ, if at all, if the patient was elderly and terminally ill; a young adult automobile accident victim; a child; or recovering well when you left the day before?

2. How would your approach differ, if at all, when providing care for the family members of a patient who died suddenly, and providing care for family members of a patient who died after a long hospitalization during which the patient wasted away and experienced pain?

CRITICAL EXPLORATION

1. Spend a day with a chronically ill child and his or her family. Record interactions and determine if any maladaptive coping behaviors are present.

2. Spend a day with a terminally ill child and his or her family. Note the family dynamics (reactions of the child and parents). Record your reaction to the situation, the child, and the family.

■ Practicing for NCLEX

MULTIPLE-CHOICE QUESTIONS

Circle the letter that corresponds to the best answer for each question.

1. Bobby, age 10, has a diagnosis of juvenile diabetes. His mother has expressed plans to tutor Bobby at home and design a comfortable, quiet life to help him cope with his condition. Which of the following nursing diagnoses would best address this situation?
   A. Readiness for enhanced parenting related to chronic illness
   B. Risk for dysfunctional grieving related to loss of child's expected activity level
   C. Risk for delayed growth and development related to lack of age-appropriate stimulation
   D. Disabled family coping related to parent's inability to accept child's illness

2. Polly, age 5, is admitted to the hospital with cystic fibrosis and pneumonia. Polly's mother tells the nurse that Polly must have pulmonary therapy before breakfast in order to eat a good meal. The nurse should respond in which of the following ways?
   A. Assure Polly's mother that the hospital staff is very competent and will take good care of the child.
   B. Inform Polly's mother of the visiting hours and insist she go home and rest since Polly is in good hands.
   C. Listen to the mother and note the schedule and procedures that Polly is accustomed to at home.
   D. Nod, and after the mother has gone plan Polly's care according to the hospital schedule.

3. Mr. and Mrs. Peters have a 4-year-old son, Bryan, who has been diagnosed with a terminal illness. The nurse would be concerned if which of the following plans were made by the family?
   A. Arrangements were being made to find a consistent sitter who could care for Bryan while Mrs. Peters works 4 hours a day.
   B. Mr. Peters states he plans to stay home with Bryan in the evenings so that Mrs. Peters can go to her exercise class.
   C. Mrs. Peters states she intends to care for Bryan around the clock and will need no assistance from anyone.
   D. The Peters family intends to take Bryan home and care for him there so he will die surrounded by family members.

4. David, 14, has leukemia and is in the hospital for the fourth time. When assessing his mother to determine if she is progressing through the stages of grief over her teenage son's terminal illness, the nurse would find which of the following to be signs of maladaptive coping?
   A. David's mother seems very sad at times and occasionally walks out of his room crying.
   B. David's mother shows the same signs of denial she showed when he was admitted to the hospital the first time.
   C. David's mother speaks of how good a son he was and how she is really going to miss him.
   D. David's mother spends a lot of time with David and brings him all his favorite foods from home.

5. The nurse notes that a terminally ill child's parents are not visiting very frequently or providing needed support. Which of the following could the nurse do?
   A. Call the parents in and have them explain to the child why they are not visiting as often as they should.
   B. Spend as much time with the child as possible, recognizing that the parents may need to withdraw temporarily to cope.
   C. Tell the child it is good to have time alone to think about death and to prepare for this new experience.
   D. Warn the parents that if they do not visit the child frequently now, they may experience intense guilt feelings after death.

ALTERNATE FORMAT QUESTIONS

Fill in the Blank

Supply the missing term or the information requested.

1. The reactions a nurse may have to the terminal illness of a child include ____________, a sense of failure and possibly all stages of grief.
2. Most school-age children ___________ what is happening to them when their disorder has a fatal prognosis.

Multiple-Answer Multiple Choice

Circle the letter(s) corresponding to the appropriate answer(s). Select all that apply.

1. Which of the following are accurate?
   A. The nurse should encourage the parents of a child in the "dying phase" to stay close to the room because the child will not live more than 2 to 3 days.
   B. The family living with a child who is dying should be provided time to talk about physical and emotional difficulties they might be having.
   C. At the onset of death, metabolism increases and the child may become flushed because cardiac stroke volume increases.
   D. Emergency drugs are best delivered intravenously as the child nears death to promote absorption and improve onset of drug action.
   E. The nurse should avoid focusing on self-awareness when preparing to work with a dying child because the focus should be on the child and family.

Answers

Chapter 1

MASTERING THE INFORMATION

MATCHING

1f, 2e, 3c, 4a, 5g, 6h, 7b, 8d

SHORT ANSWER

1. Any two of the following would be accurate: families are smaller in size; single parents are increasing in number; an increasing number of mothers work outside the home; families are more mobile, with increased number of homeless women and children; abuse is more common; families are more health-conscious; and health care must respect cost containment (see Table 1-3 in text for possible implications).
2. Nursing staff will be required to provide intensive health teaching with follow-up by home care nurses. Patients and parents must be prepared to recognize danger signs that warrant immediate attention and to respond appropriately. Parents should be allowed to do as much for the child/newborn as they wish to prepare them to care for the child/newborn upon discharge.
3. The following are methods for promoting empowerment: addressing the client by name; regarding parents as important participants in their child's health by keeping the child and parents informed of the child's status and including them in the decision-making process; and making each client feel important.

PRACTICING FOR NCLEX

MULTIPLE CHOICE

1. B 2. D 3. D 4. B 5. C

FILL IN THE BLANK

1. neonatal nurse practitioner
2. Standard

MULTIPLE-ANSWER MULTIPLE CHOICE

1. A, B, C 2. A, D

Chapter 2

MASTERING THE INFORMATION

MATCHING

1b, 2c, 3d, 4e, 5a

SHORT ANSWER

1. foster
2. communal

PRACTICING FOR NCLEX

MULTIPLE CHOICE

1. C 2. A 3. C

FILL IN THE BLANK

1. function
2. Gay or lesbian
3. Procreation

MULTIPLE-ANSWER MULTIPLE CHOICE

1. A, B, E 2. D, E

Chapter 3

MASTERING THE INFORMATION

MATCHING

1e, 2a, 3f, 4d, 5b, 6c

TRUE/FALSE

1. T 2. T

PRACTICING FOR NCLEX

MULTIPLE CHOICE

1. A 2. A 3. C

FILL IN THE BLANK

1. Hispanic
2. Chinese Americans

MULTIPLE-ANSWER MULTIPLE CHOICE

1. A, B, D, E 2. A, B, E

Chapter 4

MASTERING THE INFORMATION

MATCHING

1k, 2f, 3j, 4c, 5a, 6d, 7g, 8h, 9b, 10i, 11e

TRUE/FALSE

1. T 2. T

PRACTICING FOR NCLEX

MULTIPLE CHOICE

1. D 2. C 3. A

FILL IN THE BLANK

1. gonad
2. menopause
3. thelearche

MULTIPLE-ANSWER MULTIPLE CHOICE

1. A, B, D 2. A, C, D

Chapter 5

MASTERING THE INFORMATION

MATCHING

1d, 2c, 3a, 4b, 5e

SHORT ANSWER

1. Estrogen content of the pill suppresses follicle-stimulating hormone (FSH) and luteinizing hormone (LH). The progesterone constituent decreases the permeability of cervical mucus, limiting sperm mobility and access to the ovum. Progesterone interferes with tubal transport and endometrial proliferation, making implantation unlikely.
2. The "minipill" differs from the traditional oral contraceptive in that it is composed of progesterone only. Ovulation occurs, but implantation will not.
3. IUDs are rarely selected as a method of contraception for the adolescent girl. They are not recommended for women who have not been pregnant, who have multiple sex partners, or who are at increased risk for STIs. It is unlikely that the adolescent would fit these criteria. Spermicides and condoms, barrier methods, are commonly used by the adolescent population. They are economical and require no parental consent. However, spermicides have a conception rate of 20%. Adolescents should be cautioned carefully about the use of condoms. They are most effective when applied before any penile–vulvar contact. The self-lubricated type breaks less frequently. The condom should fit loosely enough to allow the penis tip to collect the ejaculate without undue pressure. Condom efficiency is lessened by body heat when carried for some time in pockets and wallets. The use of a vaginally inserted spermicide further enhances the efficiency of the condom.

PRACTICING FOR NCLEX

MULTIPLE CHOICE

1. B 2. A 3. B 4. B

FILL IN THE BLANK

1. Condom
2. Diaphragm

MULTIPLE-ANSWER MULTIPLE CHOICE

1. A, C, D 2. A, D, E

Chapter 6

MASTERING THE INFORMATION

MATCHING

1e, 2h, 3f, 4c, 5i, 6j, 7a, 8b, 9g, 10d

SHORT ANSWER

1. Relief; stoic acceptance; grief
2. surrogate mother
3. acidic
4. artificial insemination
5. in vitro

PRACTICING FOR NCLEX

MULTIPLE CHOICE

1. B 2. C 3. C

FILL IN THE BLANK

1. Biopsy
2. Allergic

MULTIPLE-ANSWER MULTIPLE CHOICE

1. B, C
2. A, B, D, E

Chapter 7

MASTERING THE INFORMATION

MATCHING

1d, 2h, 3f, 4b, 5g, 6a, 7i, 8e, 9c

SHORT ANSWER

1. Genetic testing allows the couple to make informed choices about future reproduction.
2. If the disease is dominantly inherited, 2 out of 4 children could inherit the disease; if the disease is recessively inherited, 1 out of 4 children could inherit the disease (see text, Figure 7-3 and 7-4).
3. Any two of the following: provide concrete, accurate information about inherited disorders; reassure people who are concerned that their children will inherit a disorder that their fears are groundless (if what they are concerned about is not an inherited disorder); allow people who are affected by inherited disorders to make informed choices about future reproduction; educate people about inherited disorders and the process of inheritance; offer support by skilled health care professionals to people who are affected by genetic illness
4. In both situations, the couple would most likely be too emotionally shocked and grief-stricken to receive genetic counseling.

PRACTICING FOR NCLEX

MULTIPLE CHOICE

1. B 2. A 3. D 4. B 5. B 6. C

FILL IN THE BLANK

1. ethical
2. inherit

MULTIPLE-ANSWER MULTIPLE CHOICE

1. A, B, C, E, F 2. B, E

Chapter 8

MASTERING THE INFORMATION

MATCHING

1d, 2h, 3j, 4b, 5f, 6i, 7a, 8g, 9e, 10c

CHRONOLOGICAL ORDER

1. End of 8 gestation weeks: Heart has septum and valves. Facial features are definitely discernible.
2. End of 12 gestation weeks: Nail beds forming on toes and fingers; tooth buds present; heart sounds audible by Doppler instrument
3. End of 16 gestation weeks: Formation of lanugo; liver and pancreas are functioning; fetus demonstrates swallowing reflex
4. End of 20 gestation weeks: Quickening experienced by the mother; beginning of vernix caseosa
5. End of 24 gestation weeks: Average weight is 550 g; passive antibody transfer from mother to fetus
6. End of 28 gestation weeks: Average weight is 1,200 g; lung alveoli begin maturing with surfactant
7. End of 32 gestation weeks: Average weight is 1,600 g; assumes delivery position; store iron
8. End of 36 gestation weeks: Additional deposits of subcutaneous fat and lanugo start to diminish

SHORT ANSWER

1. Oxygen and other nutrients such as glucose, amino acids, fatty acids, minerals, vitamins, and water diffuse from the maternal blood through the cell layers of the chorionic villi to the villi capillaries. From there, nutrients are transported back to the developing embryo. There is no direct exchange of blood between the embryo and mother; the exchange is carried out only by selective osmosis through the chorionic villi.

PRACTICING FOR NCLEX

MULTIPLE CHOICE

1. B 2. B 3. B 4. A 5. C

FILL IN THE BLANK

1. amniotic membrane
2. hydraminos

MULTIPLE-ANSWER MULTIPLE CHOICE

1. A, B, E, F 2. A, B, C, D, E

Chapter 9

MASTERING THE INFORMATION

MATCHING

1b, 2c, 3a, 4b, 5a, 6c, 7b, 8a, 9b, 10c, 11b

SHORT ANSWER

1. The nurse can play an important role in promoting health during pregnancy by providing preconception counseling and particularly by being certain that adolescents receive counseling in nutrition and safe/safer sex practices.
2. The lateral recumbent position would help prevent pressure on the vena cava that could impair circulation, and also help assist the kidneys to function at maximum efficiency.
3. The kidneys are taxed heavily to filter an increased blood volume. The glomerular filtration rate is increased, filtrating glucose faster than the renal tubules can reabsorb it, and therefore accidentally spilling glucose into the urine. In addition, lactose, the sugar of breast milk, will be spilled in the urine during pregnancy.
4. After confirmation of pregnancy, most women are more conscious about their diets, the use of over-the-counter medicines, and cigarette smoking. Also, if the woman desires to voluntarily terminate the pregnancy, the risk of complications from an abortion is minimized.

PRACTICING FOR NCLEX

MULTIPLE CHOICE

1. D 2. C 3. B 4. B 5. A

FILL IN THE BLANK

1. Multipara
2. Primigravida

MULTIPLE-ANSWER MULTIPLE CHOICE

1. A, B, C, D 2. A, B, E

Chapter 10

MASTERING THE INFORMATION

MATCHING

1b, 2c, 3a

TRUE OR FALSE

1. T 2. F 3. F 4. F 5. T

PRACTICING FOR NCLEX

MULTIPLE CHOICE

1. D 2. C 3. B 4. D 5. C

FILL IN THE BLANK

1. Gynecoid
2. Anthropoid
3. Platypelloid
4. Android

MULTIPLE-ANSWER MULTIPLE CHOICE

1. B, E

Chapter 11

MASTERING THE INFORMATION

MATCHING

1i, 2f, 3g, 4a, 5h, 6b, 7j, 8e, 9c, 10d

SHORT ANSWER

1. Education
2. Bathing: tub baths are permitted unless membranes are ruptured, cervical dilation is present, or balance is disturbed. Breast care: firm bra with wide straps, wash colostrum away with clean water, use pads inside bra to keep nipples dry and change pads frequently. Perineal hygiene: douching is contraindicated Dressing: common sense and comfort, moderate- to low-heeled shoes, avoid restrictive clothing, including garters, tight girdles, and knee-high stockings. Sexual activity: permitted as tolerated, except when membranes have ruptured or vaginal spotting is noted; if history of spontaneous abortion, refrain from sex until after the time of prior abortion; use of condom with nonmonogamous partners, use caution with oral–genital contact. Exercise: individualized, moderate activity, walking encouraged, jogging or body contact sports may be contraindicated. Sleep: increased amounts encouraged, relaxation exercises, afternoon naps in late pregnancy. Travel: no restrictions in early pregnancy, late in pregnancy arrange for emergency care in case of early labor; frequent stretching on long trips.
3. Refer to Table 11.2 of the text.
4. Refer to Box 11.6, Focus on Family Teaching, in your text; any two instructions in each category are correct.
5. Prolonged anxiety produces physiological changes leading to vasoconstriction, including constriction of the uterine vessels, which could interfere with blood and nutrient supply to the fetus.

PRACTICING FOR NCLEX

MULTIPLE CHOICE

1. B 2. A 3. B 4. A 5. C 6. C 7. B

FILL IN THE BLANK

1. teratogens
2. Radiation, hyperthermia, hypothermia

MULTIPLE-ANSWER MULTIPLE CHOICE

1. A, B, E 2. B, C, E

Chapter 12

MASTERING THE INFORMATION

MATCHING

1d, 2e, 3b, 4i, 5a, 6h, 7j, 8c, 9f, 10g

SHORT ANSWER

1. Inadequate maternal dietary intake could result in fetal deprivation with premature birth, stillbirth, functional immaturity, or congenital birth defects.
2. High parity, short intervals between pregnancies, or rigorous dieting for weight loss may deplete nutritional reserves (see text for additional factors).
3. Foods with caffeine should be avoided because caffeine stimulates the central nervous system and is associated with low birthweight. Artificial sweeteners should be avoided as much as possible, since safety is not completely established; saccharine is eliminated slowly from the fetus.
4. Protein—Source: meat, eggs, milk. Significance: supplies needed B vitamins (B12) and essential amino acids. Calcium—Source: milk, milk products. Significance: necessary for fetal skeletal and tooth formation. Fat—Source: vegetable oils are preferred. Significance: supplies essential fatty acid needed for new cell growth. Folic acid—Source: fresh fruits and vegetables. Significance: necessary for red blood cell formation. Iodine—Source: iodized salt, seafood. Significance: essential for the formation of thyroxine and proper thyroid gland function. Iron—Source: organ meats, eggs, green leafy vegetables, whole grains, enriched breads, dried fruit. Significance: needed to build hemoglobin and increased red cell volume.

PRACTICING FOR NCLEX

MULTIPLE CHOICE

1. C 2. A 3. C 4. B

FILL IN THE BLANK

1. 11.2 kg to 15.9 kg (25 to 35 lbs)
2. D; B12; calcium
3. 500, 1,000

MULTIPLE-ANSWER MULTIPLE CHOICE

1. A, D, E 2. A, C

Chapter 13

MASTERING THE INFORMATION

MATCHING

1d, 2f, 3b, 4a, 5e, 6c

SHORT ANSWER

1. A. Distraction: If brain cells of the body that register pain are all preoccupied with stimuli other than pain, these cells will not register pain. Therefore, focusing on other stimuli will divert attention and reduce pain.
   B. Reduction of anxiety: Pain impulses to the brain are enhanced in the presence of anxiety. Reducing anxiety will reduce pain perception.
2. A. Hospital settings—Advantages: Attended by skilled professionals during labor, birth, and the postpartal period; encouraged to be prepared to control the discomfort of birthing through nonmedication measures; encouraged to consider breast-feeding; emergency care and extended high-risk care are immediately available. Disadvantages: Mother does not feel totally in control of the birthing process; possible separation from the family; possible fragmentation of care.
   B. Alternative Birth Center—Advantages: Extended high-risk care is easily arranged; woman encouraged to control discomfort of labor through non-medication measures; woman encouraged to be knowledgeable about labor process and participate in decision making; woman encouraged to breast-feed; family presence; attended by skilled professionals during labor and birth. Disadvantages: extended high-risk care not immediately available; woman may be fatigued following birth and she must independently monitor her postpartal status.
   C. Home Birth—Advantages: The woman has more control over the childbirth experience and may avoid nosocomial infections; she has the greatest freedom to express her individuality and there is no separation from family; allows for family integrity. Disadvantages: adequate equipment other than first-line emergency equipment unavailable; abrupt change in goals possible if hospitalization needed; woman and support person may become exhausted due to responsibility placed on them; possible interference with "taking-in phase"; woman must independently monitor her postpartal status.

PRACTICING FOR NCLEX

MULTIPLE CHOICE

1. A 2. B 3. B

FILL IN THE BLANK

1. psychosexual method
2. effleurage
3. Kegel's
4. Gate control

MULTIPLE-ANSWER MULTIPLE CHOICE

1. B, D 2. A, D

Chapter 14

MASTERING THE INFORMATION

MATCHING

1c, 2h, 3d, 4a, 5i, 6f, 7g, 8e, 9b, 10j
1c, 2d, 3e, 4f, 5b, 6a

SHORT ANSWER

1. Refer to Box 14.1 in the textbook for examples.
2. Pregnancy results in dilated ureters and stasis of urine, which predisposes a woman to urinary tract infection.
3. Diet: 1,800- to 2,200-calorie diet, evenly distributed over three meals and three snacks. Exercise: begin exercise regimen before pregnancy, maintain consistent daily exercise, eat a protein or complex carbohydrate snack before exercise. Insulin: dosage and type may need adjustment—less early in pregnancy, more late in pregnancy. Glucose monitoring: blood testing is preferred; use milk to treat hypoglycemia.
4. Refer to Box 14.12, Focus on Family Teaching, in the text. Possible answers include: Home—do not use step stools or ladders, keep small items out of the pathway, no throw rugs, be cautious using the tub, do not overload electrical circuits, don't smoke (particularly not in bed), have good lighting when taking medications. Work—avoid toxic substances, avoid fatigue, do not stand for long periods. Auto—use seat belts at all times, do not ride with individuals who are impaired due to drugs or alcohol.
5. If victim is standing or lying down, fists should be positioned in the middle of the sternum. Pressure should be applied straight back, if victim is standing, or straight down, if victim is lying down.

PRACTICING FOR NCLEX

MULTIPLE CHOICE

1. D 2. B 3. A 4. D 5. A 6. D 7. B 8. A 9. A 10. D 11. B 12. C 13. C 14. B 15. C 16. D 17. B 18. A

FILL IN THE BLANK

1. Poor placental perfusion
2. Stasis of blood; hypercoagulability; blood vessel damage

MULTIPLE-ANSWER MULTIPLE CHOICE

1. B, D, E
2. C, E

Chapter 15

MASTERING THE INFORMATION

MATCHING

1d, 2g, 3f, 4i, 5j, 6h, 7k, 8a, 9e, 10c, 11b

IDENTIFICATION

1. C 2. A 3. B 4. C 5. B 6. A

SHORT ANSWER

1. spontaneous abortion
2. ectopic pregnancy
3. HELLP syndrome
4. mild preeclampsia
5. hydramnios
6. The time during pregnancy at which bleeding occurs helps identify the cause of the bleeding.
7. A woman with an ectopic pregnancy may experience the same initial symptoms of early pregnancy. However, if tubal rupture occurs, the woman may experience a sharp, stabbing, lower abdominal pain; vaginal spotting; and possibly signs of shock.
8. Heparin is used in DIC to stop blood coagulation so that coagulation factors will be available to restore normal clotting throughout the body.
9. A woman with multiple gestation may be instructed to do the following: maintain bedrest the last 2 to 3 months of pregnancy; refrain from coitus during the last 2 to 3 months of pregnancy; plan extra rest time during the day; eat six small meals per day instead of three large ones; report any abnormal bleeding or swelling, since the risk for eclampsia, hydramnios, placenta previa, and anemia are higher in multiple gestation. Counseling and support to help the woman work through two role changes instead of one should also be a part of the teaching plan.

PRACTICING FOR NCLEX

MULTIPLE CHOICE

1. C 2. D 3. D 4. A 5. C 6. C 7. C 8. A 9. C 10. C

FILL IN THE BLANK

1. Gestational trophoblastic disease; premature cervical dilatation
2. abruptio placentae

MULTIPLE-ANSWER MULTIPLE CHOICE

1. C, E 2. B, D

Chapter 16

MASTERING THE INFORMATION

MATCHING

1b 2a 3d 4c

SHORT ANSWER

1. privacy; confidentiality
2. leave; call; community emergency number
3. expected; they can expect
4. Nurses can encourage women to seek prenatal care and can educate women about the signs and symptoms of preterm labor so women can get help at a point at which labor can be halted.

PRACTICING FOR NCLEX

MULTIPLE CHOICE

1. B 2. C 3. D 4. A 5. D

FILL IN THE BLANK

1. family routines
2. 30

MULTIPLE-ANSWER MULTIPLE CHOICE

1. A, C, D, F, H
2. A, B, D, E, G

Chapter 17

MASTERING THE INFORMATION

MATCHING

1e, 2f, 3d, 4j, 5c, 6i, 7h, 8a, 9b, 10g

SHORT ANSWER

1. Early age of menarche in girls, an increase in the rate of sexual activity among teenagers, and a lack of knowledge of (or inability to use) contraceptive information among sexually active teenagers and desire by teens to have a baby
2. Any three of the following would be correct: pregnancy-induced hypertension, iron deficiency anemia, premature labor, preterm birth with low-birthweight infant, postpartal hemorrhage, and cephalopelvic disproportion
3. The nurse can teach adolescents about the dangers of substance abuse and the complications, both psychological and physical, of teenage pregnancy. In addition, nurses can research effective birth control measures for adolescents (that they might actually use).
4. The nurse has a legal obligation to help devise a safe plan of care for the child while protecting the cognitively challenged mother's right to maintain control of her child.
5. Any of the following would be accurate: fear of discovery and being reported to authorities for drug abuse, need for frequent drug doses and inability to wait for services, insufficient finances to support both her drug habit and medical care and nutritious food

PRACTICING FOR NCLEX

MULTIPLE CHOICE

1. A 2. C 3. B 4. A 5. A 6. A 7. D 8. D 9. A

FILL IN THE BLANK

1. emancipated minor
2. lack of engagement; prolonged; fetal descent

MULTIPLE-ANSWER MULTIPLE CHOICE

1. A, B, C, E

Chapter 18

MASTERING THE INFORMATION

MATCHING

1d, 2k, 3h, 4b, 5a, 6c, 7f, 8e, 9g, 10j, 11i

1e, 2d, 3f, 4c, 5a

SHORT ANSWER

1. temperature
2. uterus; cervix; vagina; external perineum
3. Any three of the following are correct: ripening of the cervix, increased activity level, Braxton Hicks contractions, lightening, show, and rupture of the membranes

4. Passenger; passage, powers; psyche
5. inspection; palpation; vaginal examination; fetal heart tones; sonography
6. Any three of the following would be correct: uterine muscle stretching, pressure on cervix, oxytocin stimulation, change in ratio of estrogen and progesterone, placental age and deterioration, rising fetal cortisol levels, and fetal membrane production of prostaglandin
7. Diaphoresis serves to cool and limit warming of the woman through the evaporation process.
8. Labor is longer due to ineffective descent of the fetus, ineffective dilation of the cervix, and irregular and weak uterine contractions.
9. Leopold's maneuvers are a systematic method of observation and palpation to determine fetal presentation and position. Four maneuvers are performed with the woman in a supine position with her knees flexed and her bladder empty. (Refer to Fig. 18.1 for description of each maneuver.)
10. Labor can result in emotional distress, fatigue, and fear in the woman. The nurse should provide culturally sensitive support and stress-reduction measures, promote the presence of a significant other, explain all actions, and not be judgmental or have high expectations of the woman's performance.
11. The mother's pulse and blood pressure both increase during contractions. The fetal pulse may slow slightly during contractions.
12. The father or significant other can provide an important support to the mother during the labor process and may serve as a labor coach.
13. Fetal tachycardia indicates fetal distress (severe, due to hypoxia, maternal fever, drugs, fetal arrhythmia, or maternal anemia, or hyperthyroidism). Fetal bradycardia when moderate is not considered serious and is probably due to a vagal response; if severe, it signifies fetal hypoxia. Late deceleration suggests uteroplacental insufficiency or decreased uterine blood flow during contractions. Variable pattern indicates compression of the cord. Sinusoidal pattern indicates fetal anemia or hypoxia.

PRACTICING FOR NCLEX

MULTIPLE CHOICE

1. B 2. D 3. D 4. B 5. D 6. B 7. A 8. C
9. C 10. D 11. B 12. A 13. C 14. B 15. B

FILL IN THE BLANK

1. minus (negative), plus (positive)
2. preparatory (latent)
3. ripening

MULTIPLE-ANSWER MULTIPLE CHOICE

1. B, C, E

HOT SPOT QUESTIONS

1. B 2. A

Chapter 19

MASTERING THE INFORMATION

MATCHING

1i, 2c, 3g, 4j, 5e, 6b, 7a, 8d, 9f, 10h

SHORT ANSWER

1. enduring a painful labor
2. educating women about the advantages of prepared childbirth; helping women to use breathing patterns or other comfort techniques during labor so that they need a minimum of analgesia and anesthesia; conscientious monitoring of women who receive analgesics and anesthesia during labor and birth
3. anoxia due to uterine contractions; stretching of the cervix and perineum
4. systemic; T10; L1
5. Knowledge allows the woman to make the best choices for herself and her child; it also decreases fear and anxiety related to the labor experience.
6. Knowledge reduces anxiety and decreases the amount of pain medication that may be required.
7. Pain medications given too early in the labor experience tend to slow or even stop contractions, which will delay dilation of the cervix and prolong labor. Once labor is well under way, however, pain medication could speed the progress of labor because the woman is able to work with, not against, contractions.
8. The significant other could provide support and decrease the woman's anxiety and pain.

PRACTICING FOR NCLEX

MULTIPLE CHOICE

1. B 2. B 3. C 4. A 5. C

MULTIPLE-ANSWER MULTIPLE CHOICE

1. B, C, D, E, F 2. A, C, F

Chapter 20

MASTERING THE INFORMATION

MATCHING

1b, 2c, 3d, 4a

TRUE/FALSE

1. T 2. F 3. F 4. F

FILL IN THE BLANK

1. A well-informed support person will be able to help minimize the client's experiences of anxiety.
2. A sonogram aids in locating the placenta to avoid an accidental incision of this organ during the surgical procedure.
3. Urinary output must be assessed to determine the presence of urinary retention, overextension of bladder capacity, and potential for permanent bladder damage, and to avoid interference with uterine contractions that may lead to postpartal hemorrhage. Voiding also provides evidence of adequate urinary and circulatory function.
4. Pneumonia: pain minimizes activity, allowing secretions in lung to pool. Pain increases when performing respiratory toilet exercises. Thrombophlebitis: pain discourages walking, leading to venous stasis and poor circulation of the femoral veins. Interference with maternal–infant bonding: experiences of pain lessen tactile stimulation, which hampers the bonding process.
5. Transcutaneous electrical nerve stimulation (TENS): method of controlling pain sensation by use of electrodes on the skin to irritate or stimulate the large afferent (sensory) nerve fibers, which facilitates the gating theory. The unit is turned on and off by the patient. Patient-controlled analgesia (PCA): pain control device. Patient administers precalculated dose of intravenous narcotic analgesic by pressing a button on a special pump. Pump features a "lock-out" setting to prevent drug overdose.

PRACTICING FOR NCLEX

MULTIPLE CHOICE

1. B 2. D 3. C 4. A 5. A

FILL IN THE BLANK

1. 300; 500; 500; 1,000

MULTIPLE-ANSWER MULTIPLE CHOICE

1. A, B, D

Chapter 21

MASTERING THE INFORMATION

MATCHING

1h, 2i, 3e, 4j, 5g, 6c, 7a, 8d, 9b, 10f

STAGES OF LABOR

1. A 2. A 3. B 4. B 5. A 6. A

SHORT ANSWER

1. Pathologic retraction ring; rupture
2. heart; kidney
3. cord compression; hypoxia/anoxia
4. the power (force that propels the fetus; uterine contractions); the passenger (the fetus); the passageway (the birth canal)
5. fetal monitoring and uterine monitoring
6. hypotonic uterine contractions; hypertonic uterine contractions; uncoordinated contractions
7. prolonged latent phase; prolonged deceleration phase, protracted active phase; secondary arrest of dilatation
8. small infants (SGA); cord prolapse; cord compression, intracranial hemorrhage, abnormal fetal presentation
9. dysfunctional labor, early rupture of membranes, higher risk of anoxia from prolapsed cord; traumatic injury to the aftercoming head, fracture of the spine or arm
10. occipitoposterior position; breech presentaton ; face presentation; brow presentation; transverse lie
11. woman is unable to push with contractions; cessation of progress in the second stage of labor, fetus in abnormal position, or fetus is immature
12. any two: complete, frank, double footing, single footing

PRACTICING FOR NCLEX

MULTIPLE CHOICE

1. B 2. A 3. C 4. A 5. C 6. D

FILL IN THE BLANK

1. Vaccuum extraction
2. knee-chest; Trendelenburg
3. Inertia; dysfunctional

MULTIPLE-ANSWER MULTIPLE CHOICE

1. A, C, D, F, G, H
2. B, C, E, F, H
3. B, C, D, E

Chapter 22

MASTERING THE INFORMATION

MATCHING

1f, 2i, 3c, 4d, 5a, 6h, 7b, 8j, 9e, 10g
1a, 2c, 3d, 4b

SHORT ANSWER

1. taking-in phase
2. lactation
3. episiotomy
4. During the taking-in phase the woman is passive and wishes to be ministered to; during the taking-hold phase the woman begins to initiate actions and takes more, but not all, responsibility for herself and her child; during the letting-go phase the woman redefines and assumes her new role.
5. A sitz bath supplies moist heat, which increases circulation to the perineum, thereby reducing edema, and promotes healing and comfort. An ice bag during the first 24 hours postpartum will aid in reducing edema and possible hematoma formation and promote healing and comfort.
6. Fundus: immediately postpartum, it can be found halfway between the umbilicus and symphysis pubis; it will decrease one fingerbreadth per day (1 cm/day in size) from the umbilicus until no longer palpable.

Cervix: immediately after delivery, it is soft and malleable with the internal and external os open; 7 days postpartum, the external os is narrowed to a pencil-sized opening and is firm. The external os assumes a permanent starlike or slit-like pattern.

Vagina: The hymen is permanently torn. The vagina is soft with few rugae, a large diameter, and a thin wall early postpartum. The wall may thicken and involute to prepregnancy size by 6 weeks postpartum with exercise and if proper hormone release resumes.

PRACTICING FOR NCLEX

MULTIPLE CHOICE

1. B 2. C 3. C 4. C 5. A 6. B 7. C 8. C
9. B 10. C 11. D 12. D 13. A 14. B 15. B 16. D

FILL IN THE BLANK

1. Kegel (perineal)
2. lochia serosa

MULTIPLE-ANSWER MULTIPLE CHOICE

1. A, C 2. A, B 3. A, B, E

Chapter 23

MASTERING THE INFORMATION

MATCHING

1e, 2g, 3a, 4d, 5f, 6c, 7b

TRUE/FALSE

1T, 2T, 3T, 4F

SHORT ANSWER

1. uterine atony, lacerations, retained placental fragments, and disseminated intravascular coagulation
2. deficiency in clotting, caused by low level of fibrinogen
3. premature separation of the placenta, missed early abortion, fetal death in utero
4. When wiping from back to front, organisms may be brought forward from the rectum to the vagina or perineal site of injury.
5. Assess lochia for color, odor, amount. Assess uterus for tenderness, size, and consistency. Assess vital signs to support evaluation of other data.
6. Placenta may be classed as succenturiate placenta; sections of this type may remain following a delivery and need to be surgically removed.

PRACTICING FOR NCLEX

MULTIPLE CHOICE

1. D 2. C 3. C 4. B 5. C

FILL IN THE BLANK

1. lighter
2. perineal pads

MULTIPLE-ANSWER MULTIPLE CHOICE

1. A, C, D

Chapter 24

MASTERING THE INFORMATION

MATCHING

1c, 2f, 3b, 4e, 5g, 6d, 7h, 8a, 9j, 10i

TRUE/FALSE

1. T 2. F 3. F 4. F

SHORT ANSWER

1. 30–50/minute
2. convection; conduction; radiation; evaporation
3. habituation, orientation, motor maturity, self-quieting ability, social behavior, variation
4. Bottle-fed: stools are bright yellow, have a more foul odor. Breast-fed: stools are light yellow, sweet smelling.
5. Neonates who have not passed a stool in 24 hours past birth should be evaluated for meconium ileus, imperforate anus, or bowel obstruction.
6. First period of reactivity: rapid heart beat and respiration, alert behavior, searching activity. Second period

of reactivity: occurs between 2 and 6 hours of life; baby wakes again after quiet resting period, often gagging and choking on mucus that has accumulated in the mouth. He or she is again alert and responsive and interested in the surroundings.
7. A child of 20 pounds or less should be placed with the seat facing the back of the car; car seat should have a five-point harness with broad straps; parents should not use sack sleepers or papoose clothing. Seat should face backward until the infant can sit without support (approximately 21 pounds). When the infant can sit without support, he may be transferred to a toddler car seat.
8. Hemorrhage, infection, or urethral fistula may occur.
9. Cold sores may be indicative of herpes simplex; the infant's immature immune system may render him vulnerable to a serious illness.

PRACTICING FOR NCLEX

MULTIPLE CHOICE

1. A 2. D 3. C 4. D 5. B

FILL IN THE BLANK

1. neonatal period
2. 120–140/minute

MULTIPLE-ANSWER MULTIPLE CHOICE

1. D, E

Chapter 25

MASTERING THE INFORMATION

MATCHING

1b, 2n, 3e, 4o, 5h, 6c, 7a, 8f, 9i, 10g, 11d, 12l, 13m, 14j, 15k

TRUE/FALSE

1. T
2. T
3. F
4. F
5. T
6. T
7. F
8. F

SHORT ANSWER

1. Delivery of the placenta; prolactin
2. Anterior pituitary; prolactin
3. Oxytocin; onset of labor

PRACTICING FOR NCLEX

MULTIPLE CHOICE

1. B 2. A 3. C 4. C 5. D 6. A 7. C

FILL IN THE BLANK

1. Breast; mammary
2. sucking on the breast
3. 110–120

MULTIPLE-ANSWER MULTIPLE CHOICE

1. A, C, E
2. D, E

Chapter 26

MASTERING THE INFORMATION

MATCHING

1e, 2c, 3d, 4a, 5b

TRUE/FALSE

1. T
2. T
3. F
4. F

SHORT ANSWER

1. During the first few seconds of life, infant takes several weak gasps of air and then immediately stops breathing.
2. Placenta received insufficient nutrients: partial placental separation leading to bleeding; infarction, fibrosis, and reduced placental surface for exchange. Inefficient transport of nutrients to the fetus: systemic diseases in the mother may cause decreased blood flow to the placenta. Lack of adequate nutrition: poor nutritional intake occurs in teen pregnancy.
3. Blood is removed by gravity using a venous catheter advanced into the right atrium. Blood is circulated from the catheter to the ECMO machine for oxygenation and warming, then returned to the newborn via catheter advanced through the carotid artery.
4. Periodic apnea: no bradycardia seen in the irregular breathing patterns. True apnea: irregular breathing patterns lasting more than 20 seconds with bradycardia.
5. Small plugs of meconium may be pushed farther into the lungs if infant is ventilated before the airway is cleared.
6. TTN results from slow absorption of lung fluid. Newborn respiratory rate remains between 80 and 120 after first hour of birth, mild retractions, marked cyanosis, chest x-ray reveals fluid in central lung fields with adequate aeration; syndrome peaks in 3 hours and tends to fade by 2 hours.

PRACTICING FOR NCLEX

MULTIPLE CHOICE

1. B 2. B 3. D 4. D 5. B 6. A 7. C 8. C
9. A 10.A

FILL IN THE BLANK

1. blindness, vasoconstriction
2. indirect bilirubin
3. vitamin E
4. anaerobic glycolysis

MULTIPLE-ANSWER MULTIPLE CHOICE

1. B, D, F

Chapter 27

MASTERING THE INFORMATION

MATCHING

1c, 2e, 3f, 4a, 5b, 6d
1c, 2e, 3d, 4b, 5a

SHORT ANSWER

1. Maturation
2. Growth
3. Development
4. Cognitive
5. 1. oral; infant; 1 month to 1 year
   2. anal; toddler; 1 year to 3 years
   3. genital; preschooler; 3 years to 6 years
   4. latent; school-age; 5 years to 13 years
   5. genital; adolescent; 13 years to 18 years
6. a. toddler (autonomy)
   b. adolescent (identity)
   c. school-age (industry)
   d. infant (trust)
   e. preschooler (initiative)

STAGES OF MORAL DEVELOPMENT

1. preschooler
2. adolescent (postconventional)
3. infant (prereligious)
4. toddler (punishment–obedience)
5. young school-age (conventional)

PRACTICING FOR NCLEX

MULTIPLE CHOICE

1. B 2. D 3. C 4. A 5. B 6. B 7. A 8. A

FILL IN THE BLANK

1. height, weight
2. anticipatory guidance

MULTIPLE-ANSWER MULTIPLE CHOICE

1. B, E 2. C, E

Chapter 28

MASTERING THE INFORMATION

MATCHING

1a, 2c, 3f, 4g, 5d, 6b, 7e, 8h

SHORT ANSWER

1. provides parents with opportunity to ask questions; anticipatory guidance; chart growth and development; observe for potential health problems
2. aspiration
3. ventral suspension, prone, sitting, standing, walking
4. Check sources for lead paint; use protective caps for outlets; install gates at top and bottom of stairs
5. learn different textures; provides the opportunity to kick and exercise
6. Gently wipe the teeth with cloth.
7. Change the diaper frequently, clean the area after each diaper change, and apply ointments and creams.
8. type of formula, high-protein diet, undiluted cow's milk
9. number of stools per day, color of stools, consistency of stools

PRACTICING FOR NCLEX

MULTIPLE CHOICE

1. B 2. C 3. B 4. D 5. D 6. B 7. C 8. C
9. A 10. B 11. A 12. C

FILL IN THE BLANK

1. 2 months
2. 6 months
3. yes

MULTIPLE-ANSWER MULTIPLE CHOICE

1. A, C 2. D, E

Chapter 29

MASTERING THE INFORMATION

MATCHING

1b, 2d, 3a, 4c, 5f, 6e

FILL IN THE BLANK

1. 15 months: walks alone, puts small pellets into small bottles, scribbles voluntarily with a pencil or crayon, speaks four to six words, stacks two blocks, enjoys being read to
   24 months: walks up stairs alone using both feet on same step at the same time, opens doors turning knobs, unscrews lids, speaks two-word sentences (noun/pronoun and verb), parallel play
   30 months: can jump down from chairs, makes simple lines or strokes for crosses with a pencil, can speak full name, names one color, holds up finger to show age, plays house; imitates parents, active play
2. independence

PRACTICING FOR NCLEX

MULTIPLE CHOICE

1. D 2. B 3. A 4. B 5. D 6. C

FILL IN THE BLANK

1. autonomy/independence
2. poisonings

MULTIPLE-ANSWER MULTIPLE CHOICE

1. B, C, D, G, I

Chapter 30

MASTERING THE INFORMATION

MATCHING

1e, 2c, 3a, 4b, 5d

SHORT ANSWER

1. a. large body build
   b. slim body build
   c. "knock-knee"
   d. grinding the teeth at night
2. Oedipus: preschool-age boys have strong emotional attachment for their mother. Electra: preschool-age girls have strong attachment for their fathers. Each child competes with the same-sex parent for the love and attention of the other parent.
3. Preschoolers cannot comprehend that the same procedure can be performed in two different ways. Therefore, it is important to provide continuity when caring for this age group.
4. Seek to understand the child's fears. Monitor the child's exposure to environmental stimuli that may incite fears. Use a dim light in the bedroom at night.
5. Do not ask the child to recite or sing to strangers. Do not reward or punish the child in relationship to language fluency. Listen with patience. Do not discuss the child's difficulty in his presence. See also Box 30.10 for additional information.

PRACTICING FOR NCLEX

MULTIPLE CHOICE

1. B 2. D 3. C 4. B 5. B

FILL IN THE BLANK

1. initiative
2. Oedipus complex

MULTIPLE-ANSWER MULTIPLE CHOICE

1. B, E, F, G, I, J

Chapter 31

MASTERING THE INFORMATION

MATCHING

1b, 2d, 3a, 4f, 5e, 6g, 7c

SHORT ANSWER

1. anovulatory; ovulation
2. nocturnal emissions
3. Gaining a sense of initiative is learning how to do things; doing them well is a step toward gaining a sense of industry. When a child's environment does not allow this sense of accomplishment, he develops a feeling of inferiority and becomes convinced that he cannot do many things that he in fact is able to do.
4. Decenter: ability to focus on other views besides one's own. Accommodation: ability to adapt thought processes to fit what is perceived. Conservation: ability to appreciate that a change in shape does not necessarily mean a change in size. Class inclusion: the concept that objects can belong to more than one classification (i.e., stones and shells may be gathered on the beach but they are different objects).
5. Be flexible when approving reading materials. Select readings that allow the child to complete a topic or finish in a short period of time. See also Box 31.8 for more information
6. School phobia is a child's resistance to attend school manifested by physical illnesses. The illness may be due to fear of separation from parents, fear of the younger siblings usurping the parents' love, overdependence, or overprotection by the parents. To resolve the problem, the entire family must be counseled. The parents must be

consistent and firm with the child. Initiating attendance at school gradually, such as attending school for fewer hours, may prove to be beneficial.

7. a. Drowning: Teach child to swim; advise not to try to swim beyond capabilities.
   b. Motor vehicle accidents: Encourage use of seat belts; learn to cross streets safely; learn bicycle safety rules.
   c. Sports injuries: Wear appropriate gear; do not encourage the child to play beyond his capabilities.
   d. Firearms: Teach safe use of firearms; keep firearms in locked cabinet with bullets separated from gun.

PRACTICING FOR NCLEX

MULTIPLE CHOICE

1. D 2. D 3. B 4. B

FILL IN THE BLANK

1. 9

MULTIPLE-ANSWER MULTIPLE CHOICE

1. A, B, D, E

Chapter 32

MASTERING THE INFORMATION

MATCHING

1a, 2j, 3e, 4f, 5b, 6g, 7i, 8h, 9c, 10d

SHORT ANSWER

1. mature, young
2. 13,14; 15–16; 17–20
3. formal operations; 12; 13
4. sebum formation; comedones; bacterial proliferation
5. alcohol
6. Private history-taking promotes independence and responsibility for self-care, and provides an opportunity for the youth to discuss matters he might not confide in front of a parent.
7. Inadequate diet, poor sleep patterns, busy activity schedules (also emotional problems or boredom due to understimulation)
8. Intimacy: develop intimate (close) relationships with persons of the opposite and same sex; develop a sense of compassion for other persons. Emancipation: must overcome their own and parental reluctance toward the adolescent's becoming an independent, responsible person. Value system: determine who they are, and what kind of person they want to be (must establish values of internal origin, not just mimic others).
9. Educating adolescents against cigarettes, smokeless tobacco, alcohol, drug abuse, and violence, and acting as support people for adolescents during times of crisis
10. 13-year-old: impulsive; full of self-doubt; wants to be grown-up but still looks like a child; loud and boisterous; begins to long for the opposite sex and "falls in love" for the first time. 14-year-old: quieter than at 13; more confident in self; searches for adult and older teen heroes to copy. 15-year-old: interested in approaching a member of the opposite sex; mainly physical attraction; "falls in love" frequently. 16-year-old: boys become sexually mature, though increase in height continues; both sexes are able to trust their bodies more; are more coordinated. 17-year-old: quieter and more thoughtful about interactions.
11. Any seven of the following would be correct: giving away prized possessions; organ donation questions; sudden, unexplained elevation of mood; accident proneness, carelessness, and death wishes; a statement such as "this is the last time you will see me"; decrease in verbal communication; withdrawal from peer activities or previously enjoyed events; previous suicide attempt; preference for art, music, and literature with themes of death; recent increase in personal conflicts with significant others; running away from home; inquiry about the hereafter; asking for information (supposedly for a friend) about suicide prevention and intervention; almost any sustained deviation (change) from the normal pattern of behavior

PRACTICING FOR NCLEX

MULTIPLE CHOICE

1. A 2. A 3. D 4. C 5. B 6. A 7. B 8. B 9. C 10. D

FILL IN THE BLANK

1. three
2. decrease
3. increase

MULTIPLE-ANSWER MULTIPLE CHOICE

1. A, B, F, G, I, J

Chapter 33

MASTERING THE INFORMATION

MATCHING

1d, 2c, 3b, 4a
1b, 2c, 3d, 4a

SHORT ANSWER

1. school; inspiration; expiration
2. introduction and explanation; demographic data; chief concern; history of chief concern; health and family profile; day history; past health history including pregnancy history; family health history; review of systems
3. The height and weight fall below the third percentile on a standard growth chart.
4. cover test; Hirschburg test
5. Gently press the nostril closed and ask the child to inhale.
6. The tympanic membrane may be retracted; the malleus is extremely prominent; the cone of light is missing.

PRACTICING FOR NCLEX

MULTIPLE CHOICE

1. C 2. B 3. A 4. C 5. D 6. C 7. B 8. A
9. C 10. A 11. A 12. A

FILL IN THE BLANK

1. Air
2. Geographic tongue

MULTIPLE-ANSWER MULTIPLE CHOICE

1. A, C, D, E 2. A, B

Chapter 34

MASTERING THE INFORMATION

MATCHING

1g, 2b, 3h, 4d, 5c, 6e, 7a, 8f,
1e, 2c, 3i, 4a, 5g, 6b, 7h, 8d,
9j, 10f, 11k

SHORT ANSWER

1. process recording
2. environment, family members, family functioning
3. a. psychomotor, b. cognitive, c. affective
4. redemonstration
5. type, content, time
6. physical activity
7. more economical, adds depth to learning, provides opportunity for shared experience
8. assessing the child's current level of knowledge, ability and motivation to learn new knowledge
9. Visual aids help children see and better understand what will happen and how the procedure will affect the particular body parts.
10. Children learn to a point of saturation, at which point learning stops and does not continue until that information is absorbed and understood.
11. Nurses can help by consulting with schools and health care organizations to develop health teaching programs and by teaching such programs.

PRACTICING FOR NCLEX

MULTIPLE CHOICE

1. C 2. C 3. A 4. D 5. B

FILL IN THE BLANK

1. intermixed
2. memorizing
3. stages
4. interest
5. positive

MULTIPLE-ANSWER MULTIPLE CHOICE

1. C, D, G

Chapter 35

MASTERING THE INFORMATION

MATCHING

1e, 2g, 3h, 4d, 5f, 6c, 7a, 8b

TRUE/FALSE

1. T 2. F 3. F 4. F 5. F 6. T
7. F 8. F 9. F 10. T

SHORT ANSWER

1. perception; support people; coping experiences
2. (1) harm or injury; (2) separation; (3) unknown; (4) uncertain limits; (5) loss of control
3. cognitive development; experiences; knowledge
4. stress; stress
5. favorite toy, blanket, or pacifier
6. unknown; abandonment; mutilation
7. factual
8. Children may misinterpret nursing procedures as punishments and may be confused by terms used in explanations that often sound alike or have double meanings.

PRACTICING FOR NCLEX

MULTIPLE CHOICE

1. D 2. D 3. C 4. C 5. C

FILL IN THE BLANK

1. play
2. A. infants
   B. adolescents
   C. toddlers
   D. older children/school-age
3. observation

MULTIPLE-ANSWER MULTIPLE CHOICE

1. A, D, E, F, G, J

Chapter 36

MASTERING THE INFORMATION

MATCHING

1d, 2e, 3a, 4c, 5b

SHORT ANSWER

1. clean-catch
2. obtaining an appliance small enough; skin irritation
3. Psychological preparation: familiarize the child with the techniques and equipment that are a part of the preoperative and postoperative care using an age-appropriate teaching plan. Physical preparation: nothing by mouth for a designated period of time before surgery; washing the incision area; removal of items such as barrettes and bobby pins, if present; checking the mouth for loose teeth; dressing in hospital gown and underpants; checking for correct and legible identification band
4. Any four of the following would be correct (see the text for detailed descriptions): side rails, clove-hitch, crib rails, jackets, high chairs, elbow, wheelchairs and carts, mummy (see Table 36-1)
5. Nurses can help by providing health counseling to aid in preventing children from becoming ill. Examples of actions may include preventing nosocomial infection by enforcing measures such as frequent handwashing and ensuring use of sterile technique for dressing changes. They can prevent health care worker exposure by being certain they and their coworkers follow universal precautions.

PRACTICING FOR NCLEX

1. D 2. C 3. D 4. C 5. C

FILL IN THE BLANK

1. 15
2. non-adhesive

MULTIPLE-ANSWER MULTIPLE CHOICE

1. A, C, D, E, H, L, M, N
2. A, B

Chapter 37

MASTERING THE INFORMATION

MATCHING

1e, 2d, 3a, 4c, 5b

SHORT ANSWER

1. Any four of the following: orally, intranasally, transdermally, topically, rectally, injection
2. weight, body surface area
3. intermittent infusion device (heparin lock)
4. The younger the child, the slower the rate of drug absorption, distribution, and excretion. Drugs are inactivated faster in young children than in adults but slower in newborns.
5. Restraints may be used when a child has a scalp vein infusion in place to prevent the child from touching it; a jacket restraint will help prevent the child from turning, if needed
6. automatic rate-flow infusion pump, fluid chamber, minidropper
7. right medication, right child, right dose, right time, right route, right information

PRACTICING FOR NCLEX

MULTIPLE CHOICE

1. C 2. D 3. A 4. C 5. C 6. B

FILL IN THE BLANK

1. back
2. vastus lateralis muscle
3. intravenous
4. immaturity
5. down, back

MULTIPLE-ANSWER MULTIPLE CHOICE

1. A, C, E

Chapter 38

MASTERING THE INFORMATION

MATCHING

1d, 2c, 3e, 4a, 5b

SHORT ANSWER

1. conscious sedation
2. visual analog
3. substitution of meaning

4. Any two of the following are correct: a belief that infants and young children do not experience pain; a fear of addiction to pain relief medications; a fear of causing respiratory depression
5. Pain assessment in children might be difficult because some will suffer pain rather than report it because of fear, some will distract themselves by play, and some will sleep from exhaustion caused by pain.
6. The gate control theory explains that because pain travels between the site of injury and the brain where the impulse is registered as pain, gating mechanisms in the dorsal horn of the spinal cord, when activated, can halt a pain impulse at the level of the cord.

PRACTICING FOR NCLEX

MULTIPLE CHOICE

1. A 2. B 3. C 4. B

FILL IN THE BLANK

1. topical anesthetic
2. oral analgesia

MULTIPLE-ANSWER MULTIPLE CHOICE

1. B, C, E, D, A

Chapter 39

MASTERING THE INFORMATION

MATCHING

1e, 2f, 3d, 4k, 5b, 6q, 7l, 8c, 9i, 10h, 11j, 12g, 13a, 14p, 15r, 16n, 17o, 18 m

SHORT ANSWER

1. Arnold Chiari
2. meconium plug
3. acetabular dysplasia; subluxation; dislocation

PRACTICING FOR NCLEX

MULTIPLE CHOICE

1. C 2. A 3. A 4. C 5. B 6. D

FILL IN THE BLANK

1. anencephaly
2. Ortolani's click

MULTIPLE-ANSWER MULTIPLE CHOICE

1. B, D 2. A, E

Chapter 40

MASTERING THE INFORMATION

MATCHING

1d, 2c, 3h, 4a, 5b, 6e, 7f, 8g, 9k, 10j, 11i, 12l

SHORT ANSWER

1. filter; warm; moisten/humidify
2. Any five of the following would be correct: anoxia, apnea, dyspnea, tachypnea, hypoxia, hypoxemia, hyperventilation, hypoventilation
3. A. 80 to 100 mm Hg; B. 35 to 45 mm Hg; C. 95 to 100 percent; D. 7.35 to 7.45; E. 22 to 26 mEq
4. first 24 hours; five; seven
5. frequent swallowing; clearing the throat; increasing restlessness
6. complete airway blockage
7. Any three of the following would be correct: dysphagia (difficulty swallowing), inspiratory stridor, high fever, hoarseness, sore throat, excessive drooling, protruding tongue
8. cigarette smoking; increasing activity; health maintenance

PRACTICING FOR NCLEX

MULTIPLE CHOICE

1. C 2. A 3. B 4. B 5. A 6. A 7. D 8. D 9. C 10. C

FILL IN THE BLANK

1. tachypnea
2. medulla; pons

MULTIPLE-ANSWER MULTIPLE CHOICE

1. A, C, D
2. B, D

Chapter 41

MASTERING THE INFORMATION

MATCHING

1e, 2d, 3g, 4b, 5c, 6o, 7f, 8m, 9n, 10i, 11j, 12k, 13l, 14a, 15h

SHORT ANSWER

1. left; right
2. difficulty feeding
3. air; fluid

4. hyperacute, acute, chronic
5. cardiomyopathy
6. Any three of the following are correct: bilateral congestion of ocular conjunctiva, changes in peripheral extremities, rash, swollen cervical lymph nodes, changes of mucous membrane of the upper respiratory tract such as strawberry tongue
7. medication taken during pregnancy, nutritional adequacy, radiation exposure, vaginal or other infection, cyanosis present at birth
8. information about care, steps for follow-up care and emergencies
9. use of anesthesia to induce sleep, equipment used after surgery, cough and deep-breathing exercises
10. The duration of innocent murmurs is shorter than with organic murmurs. Innocent murmurs are soft and musical; organic murmurs are harsh and blowing. Innocent murmurs are of soft intensity; organic murmurs are of loud intensity.

PRACTICING FOR NCLEX

MULTIPLE CHOICE

1. C 2. B 3. B 4. C 5. A 6. B 7. A 8. B 9. C

FILL IN THE BLANK

1. Respiratory failure
2. A. tetralogy of Fallot; B. transposition of the great arteries; C. tricuspid atresia
3. tachycardia

MULTIPLE-ANSWER MULTIPLE CHOICE

1. D, G

Chapter 42

MASTERING THE INFORMATION

MATCHING

1c, 2i, 3f, 4j, 5h, 6b, 7d, 8a, 9e, 10g

SHORT ANSWER

1. A. hypogammaglobinemia; B. IgA deficiency
2. sexual; parental
3. Autoimmunity
4. allergen
5. Reduce the child's exposure to the allergen; hyposensitize the child to produce a state of increased clinical tolerance to the allergen; modify the child's response to the allergen with a pharmacological agent
6. food diary
7. Refer to Table 42-4; any two measures in each category would be accurate.
8. Seborrheic dermatitis has no itching, onset at birth to 6 months, rarely lasts longer than 1 year, and does not cause the child to become moody. Infantile eczema causes severe itching, has a usual onset of 2 to 6 months, lasts from 2 to 3 years, and causes the child to be irritable and fussy.
9. Congential immunodeficiency disorders occur because the child is born with inadequate (or totally without) essential immune substances; secondary immunodeficiency disorders occur as a result of a loss of immunity due to factors such as infection, HIV, cancer, renal disease, malnutrition, immunosuppressive therapy, aging, or other stressors.
10. Skin testing serves to isolate the antigen/allergen to which the child is sensitive.

PRACTICING FOR NCLEX

MULTIPLE CHOICE

1. C 2. A 3. D 4. B

FILL IN THE BLANK

1. six 2. ice

MULTIPLE-ANSWER MULTIPLE CHOICE

1. A, C, D

Chapter 43

MASTERING THE INFORMATION

MATCHING

1b, 2c, 3e, 4f, 5g, 6i, 7a, 8d, 9j, 10k, 11h

SHORT ANSWER

1. viruses, bacteria, rickettsia, helminth, and fungi
2. fatal
3. 14; 21; parotitis
4. The chain of infection must be intact, consisting of a pathogen, a reservoir, a portal of exit, a means of transmission, a portal of entry, and a susceptible host.
5. Circumstances that cause a child to be susceptible to infection include a lack of natural antibodies or immunization against infection, young age, gender, the virulence of invading organisms, poor body defenses (physical, chemical), and immune type.
6. The measles vaccine may cause tuberculosis to become systemic.
7. Any time the health care worker comes in contact with bodily fluids or blood, gloves should be worn. A gown,

mask, and goggles should be worn if splattering of blood or body fluids is likely. Hands should always be washed before and after contact with clients. Sharp objects should be handled carefully. Refer to Table 42-4 in the text for reference to blood spills, specimens, and resuscitation.
8. Signs and symptoms of scarlet fever are abrupt and include fever, sore throat, headache, rash, chills, increased pulse rate, and malaise.

PRACTICING FOR NCLEX

MULTIPLE CHOICE

1. C 2. C 3. B

FILL IN THE BLANK

1. incubation
2. Rocky Mountain spotted fever
3. hookworm
4. Varicella
5. warts
6. orchitis

MULTIPLE-ANSWER MULTIPLE CHOICE

1. C, F, H, J

Chapter 44

MASTERING THE INFORMATION

MATCHING

1c, 2g, 3a, 4e, 5b, 6i, 7d, 8j, 9h, 10f

SHORT ANSWER

1. stem cell transplantation
2. hemolysis
3. graft-versus-host disease

PRACTICING FOR NCLEX

MULTIPLE CHOICE

1. B 2. A 3. D 4. D 5. C

FILL IN THE BLANK

1. platelets/thrombocytes
2. erythrocytes

MULTIPLE-ANSWER MULTIPLE CHOICE

1. A, B, F 2. B, C, D

Chapter 45

MASTERING THE INFORMATION

MATCHING

1c, 2b, 3g, 4a, 5d, 6e, 7h, 8f

SHORT ANSWER

1. gastroesophageal reflux (due to neuromuscular disturbance)
2. effortless; nonprojectile
3. dehydration; alkalosis (damage to the esophagus could also result)
4. thicker

PRACTICING FOR NCLEX

MULTIPLE CHOICE

1. A 2. B 3. B

FILL IN THE BLANK

1. Acidosis
2. Alkalosis

MULTIPLE-ANSWER MULTIPLE CHOICE

1. A, D, E, F
2. A, D, E

Chapter 46

MASTERING THE INFORMATION

MATCHING

1h, 2j, 3d, 4e, 5f, 6c, 7i, 8g, 9a, 10b

SHORT ANSWER

1. antigen-antibody
2. edema; hypoalbuminemia; hyperlipidemia; proteinuria
3. pale; oliguria; hematuria
4. The urethra is closer to the vagina in girls, and shorter and closer to the anus than in boys, allowing organisms to spread to the bladder.
5. Primary enuresis occurs if bladder training was never achieved, possibly due to mental retardation. Secondary enuresis occurs as a result of physiologic problems such as small bladder, urinary tract infection, or allergy, or psychological problems such as a new baby in the family, high stress level, change in habits, or change in environment.

6. Nephrotic syndrome occurs insidiously with rare hematuria, marked hyperlipidemia, extreme edema, and mild hypertension, whereas glomerulonephritis occurs abruptly with profuse hematuria, mild hyperlipidemia, mild edema, and marked hypertension. The treatment for nephrotic syndrome involves a high-protein, low-sodium diet, whereas glomerulonephritis commonly involves a diet normal for the age of the child; however, protein supplement or restrictions may be individually required.
7. The acute form of renal insufficiency usually occurs from a sudden body insult, whereas the chronic form of renal failure results from extensive kidney disease.
8. Salt restriction needs to be individualized: some children need less sodium, some need no restriction, and some children need additional sodium.

PRACTICING FOR NCLEX

MULTIPLE CHOICE

1. C 2. C 3. A 4. B 5. D

FILL IN THE BLANK

1. Polycystic
2. creatinine
3. Vesicoureteral reflux

MULTIPLE-ANSWER MULTIPLE CHOICE

1. B, C, E
2. A, C, D, E

Chapter 47

MASTERING THE INFORMATION

MATCHING

1f, 2j, 3c, 4h, 5k, 6b, 7d, 8g, 9i, 10e, 11a

SHORT ANSWER

1. Varicocele
2. Gynecomastia
3. Cryptorchidism

PRACTICING FOR NCLEX

MULTIPLE CHOICE

1. C 2. D 3. A 4. C 5. B

FILL IN THE BLANK

1. scrotum; rare (or painless); metastasizes
2. Mittelschmerz, abdomen
3. Balanoposthitis

MULTIPLE-ANSWER MULTIPLE CHOICE

1. A, C, D, E
2. A, B, C, E

Chapter 48

MASTERING THE INFORMATION

MATCHING

1d, 2f, 3a, 4h, 5b, 6e, 7g, 8c

SHORT ANSWER

1. insulin; glucose; hyperglycemia; ketoacidosis
2. 30
3. regulate and coordinate body systems
4. A. Thyroid gland; B. Pituitary gland; C. Pancreas; D. Pituitary gland; E. Adrenal gland; F. Pituitary gland.

PRACTICING FOR NCLEX

MULTIPLE CHOICE

1. B 2. D 3. A 4. B 5. C 6. B

FILL IN THE BLANK

1. 2; 4
2. 1–2
3. 4; 12

MULTIPLE-ANSWER MULTIPLE CHOICE

1. A, B, E
2. B, C, E

Chapter 49

MASTERING THE INFORMATION

MATCHING

1d, 2c, 3e, 4a, 5b, 6g, 7h, 8f, 9i, 10j

SHORT ANSWER

1. central; peripheral
2. balance; coordination
3. cause; expand
4. disorientation/confusion
5. arterial
6. streptococcal
7. supportive care
8. preschool

PRACTICING FOR NCLEX

MULTIPLE CHOICE

1. A 2. A 3. D 4. D 5. A 6. D 7. B 8. D 9. D 10. D

FILL IN THE BLANK

1. A. cerebellar; B. motor; C. sensory
2. A. tonic-clonic; B. simple partial; C. psychomotor; D. absence

MULTIPLE-ANSWER MULTIPLE CHOICE

1. B, C, D

Chapter 50

MASTERING THE INFORMATION

MATCHING

1h, 2i, 3f, 4g, 5e, 6b, 7j, 8d, 9a, 10c

SHORT ANSWER

1. Stereopsis
2. Orthoptics

PRACTICING FOR NCLEX

MULTIPLE CHOICE

1. B 2. A 3. C 4. B 5. D 6. C 7. A 8. A

FILL IN THE BLANK

1. Hyperopia
2. Coloboma

MULTIPLE-ANSWER MULTIPLE CHOICE

1. A, B, D

Chapter 51

MASTERING THE INFORMATION

MATCHING

1i, 2f, 3d, 4g, 5e, 6k, 7a, 8j, 9h, 10c, 11b

SHORT ANSWER

1. epiphyseal plate; periosteum
2. 1; 1.5; 20
3. thickening; enlargement; adolescent; preadolescent
4. adolescents; lift
5. 16; 3; 1; 3; 8; 12
6. The leg brace would cause the child, particularly an adolescent, to feel different from peers; the mobility limitations would also decrease opportunities for socialization with other children, resulting in isolation and decreased opportunity for development.
7. Encourage contact with school friends; arrange the bed to permit visualization of unit activities; arrange for visits from friends; maintain activity by involving the child in age-appropriate activities; tutoring may be needed.
8. Positive measures: massage the area under the cast edge with hand; apply lotion to the cast edge area; when possible blow cool air through the cast. Negative measures: avoid using coat hangers, knitting needles, or any sharp objects for scratching.
9. Walk on tiptoe for 5 to 10 minutes; practice picking up marbles with the toes; an older child could stand pigeon-toed and throw weight forward into the lateral aspect of the feet.
10. Functional scoliosis is caused by secondary physical or visual problems and is treated by correcting the underlying problem and encouraging good posture and spinal stretching exercises. Structural scoliosis is an idiopathic, often inherited, permanent spine curvature requiring long-term bracing or traction, or both. Slight curvatures may require no treatment except observation until age 18.
11. Milwaukee brace: a torso brace with one anterior and two posterior rods, leather pads, and a torso piece; used to improve spinal alignment. Halo traction: involves a metal ring attached to the skull with pins; used to stabilize cervical spine and reduce spinal curves. Bryant's traction: skin traction used for fractured femurs and for congenital developmental defects; used in children less than 2 years old. Buck's traction: skin traction used to immobilize fractured femurs in children older than 2 years old. Skeletal traction: the child's body serves as the counterpull; used to reduce dislocation and immobilize fractures.

PRACTICING FOR NCLEX

MULTIPLE CHOICE

1. B 2. C 3. C 4. C 5. B 6. B 7. C

FILL IN THE BLANK

1 rested; isometric
2 strain; sprain

MULTIPLE-ANSWER MULTIPLE CHOICE

1. B, C, D, F, G, H

Chapter 52

MASTERING THE INFORMATION

MATCHING

1b, 2j, 3g, 4c, 5a, 6h, 7k, 8e, 9f, 10d, 11i

SHORT ANSWER

1. the injuring agent; the part of the body injured; the immediate care
2. eye opening; motor; verbal
3. primary; safety precautions; children
4. Provide written instructions regarding the child's care at home; provide a telephone number for the parent to call if questions arise; schedule a return appointment for follow-up care.
5. The body proportions of infants and children differ from the adult proportions on which the rule of nines was based.
6. These burns are often accompanied by respiratory tract problems related to airway trauma due to heat, carbon monoxide, and smoke inhalation.
7. Aseptic technique and appropriate barriers are necessary to reduce the risk of infection.
8. First-degree: Cleanse the area with an antiseptic; apply an analgesic and antibiotic ointment and a gauze bandage. Do not break blister, and debride broken blisters. Keep dressings dry. Second- or third-degree: Some measures include prophylactic antibiotics; daily debridement and whirlpool; overextend joints with splints; pain management with analgesics (see toddler nursing care plan). Electrical burns: Unplug the electric cord and control bleeding with pressure to site; monitor for airway obstruction. Facial or neck burns: administer 100% oxygen; monitor for respiratory distress; prepare for tracheotomy or intubation.

PRACTICING FOR NCLEX

MULTIPLE CHOICE

1. C 2. B 3. C 4. D

FILL IN THE BLANK

1. Third
2. sterile
3. open

MULTIPLE-ANSWER MULTIPLE CHOICE

1. A, B, D, E, H
2. D, E

Chapter 53

MASTERING THE INFORMATION

MATCHING

1c, 2d, 3f, 4g, 5a, 6i, 7b, 8j, 9h, 10e

SHORT ANSWER

1. nausea; vomiting
2. induction; sanctuary (or consolidation); maintenance
3. pallor; low-grade fever; lethargy
4. node; liver
5. necessary; his life
6. compression; invasion
7. Any five of the following would be accurate: alkylating agents interfere with DNA synthesis; antibiotics impair DNA synthesis and destroy malignant cells; antimetabolites interfere with cell function; plant alkaloids interfere with cell mitosis; nitrosurea compounds interfere with DNA synthesis; enzymes remove substances needed to grow; steroids inhibit mitosis in cells; immunotherapy stimulates the immune system to attempt destruction of foreign or malignant cells.
8. Malignant cells take more than their share of nutrients from normal cells; nausea and vomiting from chemotherapy make it difficult for the child to maintain an adequate oral intake; stomatitis causes difficulty eating; and gastrointestinal ulcers and changes in fatty acid metabolism may interfere with absorption of nutrients. Some medications may alter taste sensations, which will affect appetite.

PRACTICING FOR NCLEX

MULTIPLE CHOICE

1. C 2. D 3. B 4. B 5. B 6. D 7. C

FILL IN THE BLANK

1. Ewing's sarcoma
2. Retinoblastoma
3. Enucleation

MULTIPLE-ANSWER MULTIPLE CHOICE

1. A, F, G, H

Chapter 54

MASTERING THE INFORMATION

MATCHING

1c, 2a, 3e, 4d, 5b

SHORT ANSWER

1. 1. significantly subaverage general intellectual functioning; an intelligence quotient of 70 or below with concurrent deficits; adaptive functioning
2. crying, suddenly followed immediately by giggling or laughing
3. Graphesthesia: ability to recognize a shape that has been traced on the skin; Stereognosis: ability to recognize an object by touch; Choreiform: aimless movements of arms.
4. Flat

PRACTICING FOR NCLEX

MULTIPLE CHOICE

1. C 2. A 3. B 4. C 5.D 6. B

FILL IN THE BLANK

1. pica
2. autistic

MULTIPLE-ANSWER MULTIPLE CHOICE

1. A, B

Chapter 55

MASTERING THE INFORMATION

MATCHING

1d, 2e, 3a, 4g, 5h, 6c, 7i, 8b, 9j, 10f

SHORT ANSWER

1. Special parent, different (special), special event
2. The family is a disrupted one (family members are reluctant to seek medical assistance for medical problems due to fear of discovery of abuse).
3. Abusive behavior is often the only role modeling for parenting the child has been exposed to; abuse becomes a learned behavior.
4. The nurse may tend to blame the victim due to personal feelings that somehow the abuse was deserved or provoked by the victim.
5. Place the infant on an age-appropriate diet, and if the child gains weight the problem is probably nonorganic.
6. below the third percentile for standard weight and height; motor and social developmental delays; lethargy, poor muscle tone; reluctance to initiate human contact, few comfort-seeking behaviors

PRACTICING FOR NCLEX

MULTIPLE CHOICE

1. B 2. D 3. A 4. D 5. D 6. C 7. D 8. D 9.A

FILL IN THE BLANK

1. The nurse
2. alcohol
3. repeat/support

MULTIPLE-ANSWER MULTIPLE CHOICE

1. C, D, F, H, I

Chapter 56

MASTERING THE INFORMATION

MATCHING

1c, 2e, 3b, 4a, 5d
1i, 2d, 3e, 4g, 5j, 6h, 7a, 8c, 9f, 10b

SHORT ANSWER

1. Their perception of the event, the type and kind of support they receive from people around them, and the ways they have found successful in coping with stressful situations
2. available transportation; financial situation/insurance coverage; language barriers; helpful health care providers
3. Any two of the following would be accurate: fear, feelings of failure, possibly all stages of grief
4. congenital anomalies; immunizations
5. With a nondisabling chronic illness, the child and family feel they have some control over the course of the illness. The illness would likely have minimal effect on family functioning, although some adjustments may be needed. A disabling illness will likely have a great effect on a family due to many role changes, feelings of helplessness and powerlessness, and lack of control or ability to alter the course of the disease.
6. Youth may impair the ability of parents to care for a child due to lack of experience and problem-solving ability, making all phases of parenting more difficult than for older parents. However, youth may be an advantage to parents because young parents tend to be more flexible and creative in parenting than older parents.
7. Should the child's parents die, the disabled or chronically ill child will need a designated caretaker; the will would provide for this care, should it be needed. It also would identify sources for economic support for the child.

8. Determining the effectiveness of the plan of care might help the nurse to better plan assistance for the next terminally ill child and family.
9. Any three of the following would be accurate: continue active conversation, use silence therapeutically, use the words "dying" and "death" when appropriate, preserve the dying child's defenses, sit with the child at night and allow the child to talk about dying if desired, be supportive, be aware that not all people's beliefs are the same as yours (see also Box 56.7).

PRACTICING FOR NCLEX

MULTIPLE CHOICE

1. C 2. C 3. C 4. B 5. B

FILL IN THE BLANK

1. fear
2. know/are aware of

MULTIPLE-ANSWER MULTIPLE CHOICE

1. B, D